LymeLight

LINDA WORTELL

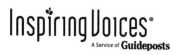

Inspiring Voices®
A Service of **Guideposts**

Inspiring Voices books may be ordered through booksellers or by contacting:

Inspiring Voices
1663 Liberty Drive
Bloomington, IN 47403
www.inspiringvoices.com
1 (866) 697-5313

ISBN: 978-1-4624-0764-4 (sc)
ISBN: 978-1-4624-0763-7 (e)

Library of Congress Control Number: 2013917928

Printed in the United States of America.

Inspiring Voices rev. date: 10/17/2013

This book is dedicated to Grace and those battling Lyme disease. Through this story, there is hope to prevent others from becoming infected with Lyme disease. A portion of the proceeds from this book will go to the John Drulle Memorial Lyme Disease Fund.

ACKNOWLEDGMENTS

Thanks be to God for His guidance throughout this journey with Lyme disease.

Thanks to my family for their support every day during Grace's illness and in writing this book. Thanks to Frank, my husband, for helping to get our family through this journey. Thanks to Michael, our son, for staying strong and supportive. Thanks to my mom for coming home to assist in providing daily help with Grace during this journey. Thanks to my dad for staying close with my son at the boarding school, so that he could achieve his goals. Thanks also to my loving friends for praying and helping in any way possible throughout our journey.

INTRODUCTION

This book is a story about our fourteen-year-old daughter's journey with Lyme disease. This disease is transmitted by deer ticks that are no bigger than the period at the end of this sentence. Once a person is infected, the infection is difficult to diagnose.

Grace's symptoms of Lyme disease were not readily recognized by the medical community. Not until Grace was seen by Lyme-literate health-care providers were her symptoms treated. Trusting in God was paramount throughout the journey. God was gracious in providing family and friends to offer advice and support whenever we needed something.

Lyme disease is preventable. I hope that what we learned and experienced on this journey, presented in this book, will prevent others from becoming infected with Lyme disease.

OCTOBER 1, 2009

"Mom how do I turn this … on?" our daughter asks, pointing to the water faucet. "How do I put on *this*?" she asks, using hand movements to mime putting on mascara. Our daughter is fourteen years old. What has happened to her? She didn't know how to turn on the water, and although she used the motions, she didn't know how to get the mascara on her eyelashes.

Imagine the chaos and confusion we experienced that morning in October 2009, when Grace woke up with sudden loss of all her long-term memory.

The day before, Grace had stayed after school for extracurricular activities and returned home like any other typical teenage girl. When you have a crisis like the one we experienced, you relive the days leading up to the event. What could have happened to cause this drastic change in our daughter? Had she been assaulted? Did she fall and hit her head? Had she been bullied? Was she drugged?

Grace, like any other American teenage girl, had gone to middle school at seven o'clock in the morning on the day before this strange chain of events. After school, our neighbor picked her up from color-guard practice, and she got home at five. She'd had a long ten-hour day at school and extracurricular activities, but this was typical of her everyday schedule. When she arrived home, everything was normal. After eating a healthy dinner, she proceeded up to her room to do her homework. Again, everything was normal—physically, psychologically, and socially. Grace did not complain of feeling sick. She did not talk about anything upsetting her.

Later that evening, Grace asked me to quiz her on the science material in preparation for a quiz for the following week. With clarity, she verbalized her knowledge of the material. Grace still had several days to review and master a few remaining study-guide items. I was impressed with her knowledge of this subject. As Grace went to bed, she had a runny nose, and I gave her a decongestant before she fell asleep.

Never in my mind did I anticipate how our lives would change in eight hours. These were the last eight hours of pure sleep and relaxation we would have for many months. When Grace awoke the next morning, it was instantly apparent something was wrong. Grace's speech was not clear as she woke up. The words she spoke were clear but nonsensical. She was talking about things as if she had woken from a deep sleep. Grace finally got out of bed and walked into the bathroom, her normal routine in the morning before school. I went down to the kitchen to prepare breakfast and lunch for the day ahead. I would be leaving for work as Grace left for school.

Grace came downstairs into the kitchen, complained of a headache, and was asking how to do things that are simple and natural for a teenage girl.

I am a nurse, but I didn't suspect anything was seriously wrong; I thought Grace just needed to eat. I gave her Tylenol for her headache and said, "Let's sit down and have breakfast."

I thought, *Let's relax and regroup, and we'll get going in a little bit.* Even though we might be later than normal, we would get our day together. I've always been a mother who goes with what God has given me to work with. So being late this morning would not be a huge deal. We could only do what we could do.

As Grace and I sat to eat breakfast, I ate one spoonful of oatmeal and then dropped my spoon as I watched my daughter. Grace didn't know what to do with the cereal in front of her or how to use a spoon. I thought, *Oh Lord, Grace is having a stroke.* What else could it be? A fourteen-year-old just doesn't forget how to eat.

I knew that prompt medical attention improves recovery for stroke victims, according to all of the current medical literature and protocols. Immediately, Grace and I left for the local community hospital. Yes, this was the right thing to do. A stroke was life-threatening but caught in the early stages, the prognosis would be much better. We left so abruptly, I did not wake up my husband to tell him about the situation. Time was of the essence. I planned to call him from the emergency room.

I recalled a young boy in our community who had suffered a stroke the year before. As this young boy got off the school bus at the end of a school day, he experienced weakness and confusion. His mother was able to get him to the local hospital for immediate medical attention. His recovery was 100 percent. So our going to the hospital was imperative.

We would do whatever we had to do to get through this. Praying for strength to hold us together was all that we had at that time, as God carried us.

The day we had planned was indeed not what God had planned for Grace and me. I quickly realized I would not be able to teach my nursing students on this day as scheduled, but how could I get that information to the students at this late notice? I placed a call to one of my nursing students and asked her to inform my class I wouldn't be there. I told her, "Something is wrong with Grace, and I must take her to the emergency room."

I then left with Grace for fifteen-minute drive to the hospital. Later in Grace's illness, the short distance to this local hospital would seem like a journey across the entire state of Pennsylvania. We would travel this route with continuous prayers for comfort and healing.

Upon arrival at the hospital, Grace was triaged immediately and seen by nurses and physicians within minutes.

The first nurse to see Grace asked, "What is your name and your birthday?" As a nurse, I know nurses do this to verify who the patient is and to assure proper treatment is given to the correct patient.

Grace just stared at the nurse.

The nurse looked toward me with a slightly irritated expression.

I quickly responded, "She doesn't remember anything. That's why she's here." I followed up by providing the nurse with Grace's name and birthday.

Quickly, the nurse placed an armband on Grace and moved her into an emergency room examination room.

Immediately, another nurse entered the examination room and introduced herself. She asked, "What is your name and your birthday?"

Again, Grace stared at her and then looked to me.

I anxiously stated, "She can't remember anything. That's why she's here." My heart was pounding, and my voice began to quiver. "Oh Lord, they do not know how desperate we are. Please show them," I prayed, whispering prayers to God.

The emergency room physician came into the examination room while the nurse was still gathering information. He introduced himself and asked Grace, "What is your name?"

For the third time, I explained Grace did not know her name, birthday ... or anything.

The physician and nurse had the same body language at that moment, one that seemed to say, "There is no way this teenage girl doesn't remember anything."

The nurse asked Grace to count to twenty.

Grace very slowly said, "One ... two ... three ..." Then she stopped. Grace didn't know the next number. She looked at me with tears—and questions—in her eyes.

Being thorough, the nurse continued to gather assessment information by asking Grace to say the alphabet.

Grace had no response at all, other than to glance at me again with bewilderment in her eyes.

Next, the nurse pointed to me and asked Grace, "Do you know who this is?"

Very quietly, Grace smiled and said in a childlike voice, "Mom."

I smiled with relief. Praise the Lord; she knew me as Mom. But why was the rest of her memory gone?

The nurse continued, "Do you have any brothers or sisters?"

Grace glanced at me and shrugged her shoulders.

That morning, I had put on a sweatshirt with "Culver" written on it. This was the name of the boarding school our son attended. I pointed to the name on the sweatshirt and said, "Your brother, Michael, goes to school at Culver."

None of this made any sense to Grace. Her look of bewilderment would be a distinct memory of these days. Grace had just seen her brother ten days earlier, yet she didn't know if she had a brother—or even what a brother was.

How was it possible that Grace could remember me, her mother, and no one else? Through God's grace, she remembered the one person who would not only be her mother but her caregiver and advocate for each remaining day of this ordeal.

Now, the nurse and physician came to the same conclusion I had— this was a stroke. A CAT scan and blood work would confirm the stroke, and prompt attention would minimize the complications of the stroke.

The nurse continued to ask Grace more questions. "Are you pregnant?"

Grace responded with a stare that indicated she didn't understand.

The nurse then asked, "Did you take any drugs?"

Grace adamantly said, "No."

"Did anybody give you any drugs?" the nurse asked.

Again, Grace adamantly said, "No." Tears welled in her eyes.

The nurse left the examination room to gather supplies for blood work to test for drugs and pregnancy. As the nurse left the room, Grace quietly stated, "I'm not like that." Somehow, Grace was able to assert her personality and character, even though she didn't have her memory. She understood the connotation of drugs as being something she would not do. I reassured Grace that everything had to be tested to figure out what had happened.

Vial after vial of blood was drawn. Then, the nurse tried to insert an intravenous line. She was unsuccessful and called in another nurse to get the IV started. This was another nurse to ask simple questions to which Grace didn't have the answers.

The cycle repeated itself. The nurse asked, "What is your name and your birthday?"

Grace had no response, so I answered the questions again. *Lord, please provide me with strength and patience as we seek a diagnosis for Grace.*

I tried to guide Grace through the procedures, step-by-step. I explained who the people were and what things meant. I waited outside of the room where the CAT scan was being done, as I was not allowed in due to the radiation. The flashing lights and loud noises of the

CAT scan scared Grace more than anything else did that morning. Grace continued to complain of a severe headache and light and noise sensitivity. The CAT scan was almost more than she could bear at that time in her illness. However, I knew that the CAT scan would provide a diagnosis for her condition.

Grace was taken back to the ER examining room. Within fifteen minutes, the ER physician came into the room to tell us the CAT scan did not indicate a stroke. *Oh Lord, the CAT scan does not indicate a stroke. What is happening? Is it meningitis? Is it encephalitis?*

The emergency room physician discussed these other possible diagnoses with me and suggested a lumbar puncture to rule out these central nervous system infections. I consented to the procedure for Grace. She tolerated this procedure better than the CAT scan. *Surely,* I thought, *this will confirm a diagnosis, and treatment will begin.* Prompt treatment seemed essential to treat the sudden onset of memory loss and to stop any further damage from occurring.

By now, Grace and I had been in the emergency room for approximately an hour. There was a period of calm after the tests were performed, and we were left to wait for results. I knew in my heart that a diagnosis would be made once the laboratory had the results.

I took the time to place a few very difficult phone calls. First, I called my husband, Frank, Grace's dad. He was home sleeping when we left the house. He was a pilot and had to fly a domestic flight later in the day. I left him a message on the home phone and cell phone. Second, I called my parents, who lived in Indiana near our son's boarding school, seven hundred miles from our home in Pennsylvania. My parents had agreed to spend the school year in the vicinity of our son's boarding school to support him and his new friends during their schooling. I desperately tried to be brave as I gave my parents the details of the morning so far and let them know we were waiting for results. We surely would have answers soon. Next, I called and left a message for Angela, our "angel," the leader of our Bible study, which would be meeting within an hour for the weekly study.

After this quiet period, the emergency room physician came into the room. "All of the lab work came back negative," he informed me.

I'd had experiences like this before, when I hoped a physician would make a diagnosis when one of my children was sick, because then there would be a medical protocol rather than "wait and see." Now, it would have been better to have a medical diagnosis. If it was a stroke, a protocol would be followed, and her symptoms would improve. If it was encephalitis or meningitis, there would be a medical protocol to follow.

Assessing Grace's day before this episode was leading to dead ends for the health-care professionals. Grace couldn't remember what happened at school the day before. She couldn't count past the number three. She couldn't say the alphabet. She didn't know the names of colors. Had she fallen? What had happened? These would be questions that were unanswered.

After we learned the tests were negative, my husband, Frank, came to the emergency room. As he approached Grace's bed, Grace whispered to me, "Who is that?" This was heartbreaking. How could our daughter not know her father?

He greeted Grace with his usual jovialness. "Hey, how are you doing?"

Grace shrugged and looked toward me.

I quickly gave him an update on the events and tests. He was as bewildered as Grace, yet he seemed to think the doctors would figure this out.

During the assessment, we realized Grace did not know anybody, except for me. I even went to the car to get a picture of our son to show Grace. I was thinking if she could see his picture, she would remember him. She had always been particularly close to her brother. The picture, however, only further confused her. I had been the last person with her prior to her memory loss. Thank God she had somebody in her memory to help her through this journey. Unfortunately, Frank needed to leave for work as we waited for further information. We agreed he could go to work and be in contact throughout his trip, as there would surely be a prompt diagnosis and treatment. I prayed for guidance as I faced the daunting medical system with my daughter alone.

Within an hour, Angela and another Bible study friend, Heidi, came to the ER to offer spiritual support. These two ladies were close to our family. As they approached Grace's bedside, Grace again whispered, "Who are they?" Before this morning, Grace would have readily recognized and talked to them.

I pointed to Angela and quietly explained to my daughter, "That is Angela. She is our friend at Bible study." Then I pointed to Heidi and continued calmly, "That is Heidi. She is another friend of ours from Bible study."

Grace smiled shyly and looked toward our friends.

I am blessed and amazed that Angela and Heidi were at Grace's bedside. I'd thought they were having Bible study. Throughout our discussion, they stated their call from God to come and be at Grace's bedside. I provided them with a summary of the details of the morning so far. We prayed at Grace's bedside for the health-care professionals who were treating Grace, for Grace, and for our strength and patience during this difficult time.

Angela helped me to think through possible contributing factors to this bizarre situation. She stated, "Did you tell them about her Lyme disease?" Angela had Lyme disease in the past and recalled Grace had Lyme disease two months earlier.

Lyme disease is a bacterial infection spread by deer ticks. A person infected with Lyme disease may experience flu-like symptoms, including body aches, low-grade fever, and stiff neck. If Lyme disease is undiagnosed or undertreated, further symptoms may develop, such as arthritis, severe headaches, Bell's palsy, and short-term memory loss. Angela and I hoped and prayed to connect Grace's current symptoms with the known symptoms of Lyme disease.

The next time the physician came into the examination room, I stated that Grace had been diagnosed and treated for Lyme disease in August, just two months earlier. He wrote the information on the chart. We couldn't come up with any other missing details for the health-care professionals.

After only four hours in the emergency room, Grace's nurse chatted with me as a mother and as a fellow nurse. "The doctor is going to discharge her," she said.

My mind was whirling. *Why?* I thought. *How could this be?* We didn't have any answers. My fourteen-year-old daughter had sudden long-term memory loss, a severe headache, and noise and light sensitivity, and she was going to be discharged.

Through our discussion, the nurse said, "When you can't handle this anymore, you should go to the Children's Hospital." It was about thirty miles away.

We live in the United States of America. We have superior health care. How could they discharge us with no direction and no answers? This was unbelievable. I have been a registered nurse for twenty-five years. I would never have believed this could happen.

My two Bible study friends traveled home with me to regroup before leaving with me for the Children's Hospital in Philadelphia. We needed to go to our home first to let the dogs out for a little bit and put on comfortable clothes for what we felt would be a long day ahead of us. Also, we packed an overnight bag, as I felt we surely would be staying at the Children's Hospital while Grace received treatment.

As we went into our house, where we had lived for seven years, I directed Grace to go upstairs to her bedroom. "Get your yoga pants," I said.

Grace stood beside me and said, "Where is my bedroom? And what are yoga pants?"

I took a very deep breath and went as calmly as possible to Grace's bedroom with her. I explained to Grace, "This is your bedroom. I am getting your yoga pants because they will be comfortable." Grace followed me closely as I moved around her bedroom, gathering the items I felt we would need at the Children's Hospital.

Angela, bless her heart, cleared any obligations she had for the remainder of the day so that she could be with Grace and me. Heidi offered to come over and watch our dogs during our time at the Children's Hospital. I appreciated both of them for giving their time and love to help us through this day.

Once in the car, I drove carefully for the hour it took to get to the Children's Hospital. I avoided quick stops and as many bumps in the road as possible. This was to avoid inflicting Grace with anymore stimulus and intensifying her severe headache. Grace rode quietly, occasionally peering out from under the blanket into the broad daylight.

Angela and I told her things as we drove, such as what the buildings were, where we were, and how much longer it would be until we arrived. Nothing appeared familiar to Grace at all. Her eyes were filled with bewilderment. Angela and I exchanged glances and prayerful thoughts.

This was not the first drive to Philadelphia for Grace. As a family, we go into the city several times a year for cultural events, the theater, and field trips, although none of this road was a retrievable memory at this time for Grace.

Angela and I prayed often and supported Grace through her pain and confusion. By the time we arrived at the Children's Hospital emergency room and Grace was triaged into an emergency room cubicle, it was late afternoon.

The first resident to assess Grace asked routine questions—"What is wrong?" and "How long has this been going on?" I answered the questions for Grace and provided a concise history of Grace's current condition, as we reviewed the data from the first hospital. I mentioned that Grace had been diagnosed with Lyme disease two months earlier. The resident noted the details in the medical record without any perceived level of alarm.

Angela and I continued to wonder if Grace's condition was related to Lyme disease.

"Is Grace's severe headache related to Lyme disease?" I asked. "Is it possible that her memory loss is related to Lyme disease?" Short-term memory loss is a noted symptom of Lyme disease, but Grace had lost her long-term memory.

This resident didn't seem to connect these symptoms to Lyme disease. He prescribed medicines to reduce the headache pain, to be given through an intravenous line. He reviewed the CAT scan and laboratory information that I'd brought from the first hospital.

The resident asked questions—"Who is the president?" and "What day is it?"—which Grace couldn't answer. These were questions met with blank stares and responses of "I don't know."

The nursing staff was caring and helpful. The nurses spoke softly to Grace and limited the stimulus to try to alleviate her headache.

The resident returned to assess Grace's headache pain and said she could eat. Since it was now approaching six o'clock, the neurology team had already left for the day.

"How can a large teaching hospital for children not have a neurology team on staff twenty-four hours per day?" I wondered out loud.

"The neurology team would come back to the hospital if there was an emergency," the resident said, "but otherwise, they are not available."

Is this not an emergency? I thought. *My daughter has a severe, debilitating headache and suddenly loss of her long-term memory. What part of this is not an emergency? Are seizures and strokes the only emergencies that would warrant the neurology staff's return to the hospital? What rights do I have as the mother of this patient? Can I not demand she be seen by a neurologist?*

Bewilderment set in. Couldn't anyone see this was a crisis? We came to this hospital for answers. We came here for some treatment. Wasn't there anything somebody could do to help with the sudden memory loss? They focused on the pain, but the memory loss was just as important, if not more important.

Grace's headache had improved slightly with the intravenous medication. She had not eaten anything all day except for a muffin. Maybe once she got some food in her system, she would begin to improve. Angela agreed to sit with Grace while I got some food. "What would you like to eat?" I asked.

Grace didn't know any foods; she didn't remember. I would do my best to bring back things she enjoyed before today. While I was gone from the room, Angela and Grace discussed sandwiches—different things that go on sandwiches and different things one eats with sandwiches, such as chips and fries. Angela was trying to find some familiar memories to work.

I brought back a variety of food, all of which were new memories to Grace. She enjoyed learning what ravioli was. She learned how to use a spoon to feed herself. She stated the ravioli was "delicious," using the word appropriately. She learned how to drink from a straw, which she enjoyed. Overall, Grace tolerated eating and did not feel any nausea, although her headache did not change.

As we sat through the evening hours, we prayed and taught Grace what we could about her surroundings. Several hours passed without any further diagnostic procedures or interventions. The medication continued to infuse through her intravenous line, and an occasional nurse or resident came to check on Grace's headache. Nothing was being done about her memory loss.

Grace was discharged shortly before midnight—we'd been there seven hours. I recall saying to the attending physician, "You are sending me home without any treatment. What do you expect to happen?"

She replied, "Grace's memory will come back over time." The resident provided no explanation of why Grace's memory had gone away. The resident provided no information on what to expect or when to expect it.

The only thing we were given was a prescription for a medication to help Grace with her headache. We were also told that the neurology staff would contact us in three business days to make an appointment to see Grace.

Truly, we were in God's hands. No human was able to help us at this time. Seventeen hours after Grace was first seen in an emergency room, we were headed home to face any issues on our own—with God's help. The footprints were definitely in the sand.

Imagine, for just a few moments, having a loved one lose her entire memory and after two emergency room visits over seventeen hours, she is discharged without a diagnosis or a treatment plan. What would you do? Now, imagine being at home alone with your loved one with no answers and no treatment plan.

Three business days! Then we would get a call to make an appointment. Unfortunately, the day that Grace's memory was lost was a Thursday. I could expect a phone call to make an appointment on Tuesday of the following week! Grace had no memory, severe headaches, and light sensitivity and noise sensitivity. What would we do? How would we survive? When would there be answers?

Our only discharge instruction was to wait for Grace to improve. She would improve "with time." We would just have to wait.

God was our only hope. We prayed for guidance through this unbelievable experience. Prayers became the support to endure the upcoming days. Prayers were offered for my own well-being as my daughter's sole care provider at this time. Prayers, prayers, and prayers.

> *Even though I walk through the*
> *Darkest valley,*
> *I fear no evil;*
> *For you are with me;*
> *Your rod and your staff-*
> *They comfort me.—Psalm 23:4*
> *New Oxford Annotated Bible;*
> *Oxford University Press 1994*

THE NEXT TWO WEEKS

So you have pain now; but I will see you again, and your hearts
will rejoice, and no one will take your joy from you.—John 16:22
New Oxford Annotated Bible; Oxford University Press 1994

Frequently, I updated my faithful friends and family through e-mails, and they graciously and willingly offered to help in any way. Through God, they were with me throughout this journey and truly were my blessing.

The morning after Grace's sudden memory loss, I let her sleep late because the previous day had been so long and painful, physically and psychologically. As I woke her up, I offered, "I will make you whatever you want for breakfast."

"What is breakfast?" Grace asked.

"For breakfast, you like pancakes or French toast," I informed Grace.

"What are pancakes?"

I trembled as I spoke. "How about if you come down to the kitchen, and I will show you?"

Grace had always loved to cook and dreamed of pursuing culinary arts in her future. Now, when she came down to the kitchen, she opened each and every drawer and cabinet, pulling items out and asking what each one was with a sad look on her face. She had a severe headache and couldn't stand the bright sunshine coming in the kitchen window.

As she sat down to eat breakfast, I nearly lost my composure. I mixed up pancake batter and thought Grace would come over to the stove to cook the pancakes. Instead, she sat staring at me. I cooked the pancakes and placed them on a plate in front of her with syrup. Grace didn't know how to use a fork and a knife. What was I to do? Home alone, I prayed for guidance and for support. I felt the embrace of God's arms and knew I wasn't alone.

I quietly showed Grace how to hold a fork and a knife. Then I taught her how to cut with the knife. This did not come easily. She simply pushed down with the knife, rather than sawing back and forth. Grace ate her breakfast and then quickly lay down on the sofa in the darkened family room because of her severe headache and light sensitivity.

Something else was missing from Grace's life. She had no appetite at all. I didn't know if this was due to the severe headache or something else. She didn't have an aversion to any foods; she simply had no appetite. She didn't remember her favorite foods. She didn't know which foods to eat at different meals. Everything was new to her.

As Grace lay quietly on the sofa, I had to take care of the human aspect of this situation. As a mother and as a nurse, I had to come up with a plan. I continued to wonder, *How could I be sent home to wait with no answers?*

I sat on the deck in the back of our house to keep the house quiet for Grace. I thought she might fall asleep while I made the phone call to the Children's Hospital neurology staff office. I felt there must be a way to get the appointment made today. I am not a person to sit and wait for things to come together. I would take steps and get closer to a diagnosis for Grace. When I called, however, I was told by the neurology office secretary that the person to make the appointments was not in the office.

"This is unbelievable," I said loudly as I hung up the phone. I sat there and cried. I asked God to please show me the way.

Although I'd hoped to speed things along, we were forced to spend the weekend without a diagnosis and without a treatment plan. Grace and I lived in our basement, away from noise and light and any other stimuli for the duration of the weekend. Still, I felt I must come up with a plan to get through this incredible situation. Frank returned from his trip on Saturday, and we developed an action plan: return with Grace to the emergency room at the Children's Hospital on Monday morning and wait until the neurology team saw our daughter. All we needed to do was to be patient and courageous until then. Surely, on Monday, four days into her memory loss, she would be assessed by the neurology team, and she would get some relief, some answers, and some direction.

The weekend seemed endless. The only time Grace and I came out of the basement was to use the bathroom. I quickly prepared snacks and brought them down to Grace periodically. Watching the television was impossible, as the light bothered Grace and worsened her severe headache. Grace did not remember how to play any board games or card games. She didn't want to look at photo albums, as she was unable to focus. So we quietly chatted and enjoyed visits from a few friends. Angela brought a goodie bag with a soft fleece blanket that Grace snuggled in.

We prayed often for peace and relief. "What else can we do except wait?" I asked God frequently during the weekend. One good sign I observed during the weekend was that as I retaught Grace things, such as how to drink through a straw, she was able to remember later that day and on subsequent days.

Grace's severe headaches continued for the weekend. After a very painful and stressful weekend, my husband and I took Grace to the Children's Hospital emergency room on Monday, where Grace was triaged into an examination room. We provided the details of the past four days to the resident, stressing Grace's memory loss and severe headaches. In Grace's medical history questions, we included her diagnosis of Lyme disease two months earlier.

The resident and the neurology team began examining Grace. The physicians badgered her with questions.

"What do you use a hammer for?"

"I don't know," Grace blankly stated.

"How do you light a candle?"

"I don't know," Grace stated again.

"Show me how to tie your shoe."

Grace stared at me.

"What is your favorite color?"

"I don't know," Grace repeated.

"What do you like to eat?"

Grace remained silent.

Grace's responses to the questions seemed defiant. Her lack of response and "I don't know" were consistent throughout the whole assessment.

After a thorough assessment, the neurology team left the examination room. We watched as the neurology team stood at the nurses' station discussing the matter for at least twenty minutes. Frank and I anticipated that they would come back with a diagnosis and a treatment plan. We believed answers would be forthcoming. Praise the Lord.

The chief of neurology returned to Grace's bedside and informed us that they could not find anything physically abnormal with Grace. Therefore, he insisted, "This must be a psychiatric issue." He described his proposed treatment plan: admit Grace to the psychiatric unit to be further evaluated and treated.

In reality, we knew parents tend to deny their children have a problem, whether physical or psychological. Parents often have their protective blinders on when it comes to their own children. Their sweet, innocent children are perfect in their eyes. Parents of teenagers have a difficult task in raising responsible teenagers in this society. I realized that Grace had been at school for ten hours on the day before her sudden long-term memory loss and severe headache. I personally did not know what she had experienced that day—but neither did Grace. She couldn't tell any of us that somebody had bullied her or if she had fallen and hit her head. She could not remember.

Stop! I screamed to myself with terror in my eyes. *What was this chief of neurology saying to us?*

The chief of neurology wanted to admit our daughter for a psychiatric evaluation and treatment. It was possible that Grace had suffered a traumatic event, but to leave her in Philadelphia in the psychiatric unit was not something I felt led to do. God's guiding hand was with me at this crucial moment.

I quietly asked, "What are our other options?"

With hesitation, the chief of neurology offered, "You could get outpatient psychiatric care for Grace."

"How do we get that set up?" I asked.

"I will send a social worker in to make the arrangements for you," he responded.

After the chief of neurology left the examination room, my husband commented, "Maybe we should consider having Grace treated here."

I explained that she would likely only have an hour of therapy a day. "Why should we leave her here with all of these strangers? She can have therapy closer to home."

Within a half an hour, a social worker came to discuss outpatient psychiatric care. She politely asked Frank and me to leave the examination room while she talked with Grace by herself. She asked our daughter questions regarding physical abuse, and we were not allowed to be in the room at that time. After this questioning, the social worker asked us to come back in the room. At this time, she discussed the option of outpatient psychiatric care. I promptly supported the decision to have Grace be at home and be evaluated and treated locally. My husband was in agreement with the treatment plan.

Upon discharge the second time from the Children's Hospital, the treatment plan was not easily implemented. We were instructed to consult Grace's pediatrician for a referral to a local psychiatrist. Even though the Children's Hospital had outpatient centers within twenty miles of our home, they were unable to refer us to a local psychiatrist. I spent the next day calling the pediatrician and explaining this step in our journey and getting the name of a psychiatrist.

Twenty-four hours after Grace was discharged from the hospital emergency department, I was able to speak to a psychiatrist on the phone about Grace's condition and diagnostic evaluation so far. Throughout our thirty-minute telephone conversation, the psychiatrist gathered information about Grace's sudden memory loss and severe headaches. In the discussion, I included the details of the three hospital visits and the lack of a diagnosis or treatment plan to date. He described the plan to further rule out any physical reasons for the memory loss and severe headaches. He was precise and confident in describing his action plan to me that evening.

Within two more days, the psychiatrist saw Grace and evaluated her and our family unit. After an hour evaluation, the psychiatrist described the diagnostic process, which would attempt to rule out anything physically abnormal with Grace. The psychiatrist ordered an EEG and an MRI to further eliminate any physical abnormality leading to Grace's memory loss. If no physical cause of the severe headaches and memory loss could be found, she would likely be diagnosed as having a conversion disorder. The psychiatrist explained the diagnosis was used when symptoms such as memory loss couldn't be explained by medical diagnoses; it was a mental health disorder.

In order to schedule the MRI and the EEG, the insurance company needed to approve these diagnostic tests. Within a few days, we received the approval from the insurance company. I immediately scheduled the MRI and EEG for the earliest dates available. Unfortunately, we still had to wait for ten days for the tests.

One more step would be necessary before the MRI. Grace's orthodontic braces needed to be removed. The magnetic field in the MRI would pull on the metal of her braces. No metal of any kind is allowed in an MRI. So I promptly scheduled an appointment with Grace's orthodontist, who compassionately arranged to come into the office during off-hours to provide a quiet environment for Grace, decreasing the stimuli.

The reality set in that there was not going to be an easy answer or any quick treatment for Grace's severe headaches and memory loss. To manage everyday life, I arranged "kid-sitters" to be with Grace. My faithful Bible study friends and neighbors offered to help in any way. I listed each of their names, phone numbers, and the days they were available on a pad of paper. This became my support to manage Grace's care and to continue teaching nursing students two days per week. I knew early in the journey that maintaining normalcy might benefit Grace as well as me.

Also, we asked friends and family not to phone us. By this point, it was overwhelming to have a phone conversation with one person about the most recent information and then to hang up and have another call from a concerned family or friend. I emotionally could not handle telling the details frequently. I deeply appreciated everybody's concern, love, and prayers, so I established an e-mail group and sent out daily updates. Through this, my friends and family could easily send a prayer or thought to us without the anxiety of each phone call. Plus, I needed the time to care for Grace rather than talking on the phone.

One afternoon, our priest and his wife stopped by for a short visit. As they walked in the door, Grace looked at me for information. She was totally lost. I quickly explained to Marshall and Laura, "Grace does not remember who you are." Marshall was always jovial and personable, and he sat down beside Grace and chatted with her as a caring friend. Grace was pleasant and accepting of our friends, even though she did not know them.

Marshall and Laura brought a bag of cider doughnuts for Grace. As they handed the bag to Grace, I explained to her, "Those are doughnuts. Try a bite and see if you like them."

Marshall and Laura saw firsthand the impact of Grace's memory loss. Laura's face saddened as she quietly sat across the room from Grace.

We were facing another weekend before any further appointments. Grace continued to have total memory loss and severe headaches. Rather than sit at home for the weekend, Frank and I decided to travel to see our son, Michael, at boarding school. This was an opportunity to reintroduce Grace to her brother and her grandparents.

OCTOBER 16-19, 2009

God, grant me the serenity to accept the things I cannot change;
The courage to change the things I can,
And the wisdom to know the difference.
Amen.

Two weeks into Grace's journey, we all traveled to see our son and my parents. It was an eleven-hour car ride that we had made numerous times during the prior school year. Grace still did not remember her brother, her grandmother, or her grandfather. On the drive, my husband and I retaught Grace many things during the day of traveling. Our main focus was to manage Grace's headaches as best as we could during this all-day car trip. *Staying at home wouldn't have been any better,* we thought. Plus, a part of us was praying for Grace's memory of her brother and grandparents to return as she met them.

Halfway through the drive, I profoundly realized the intensity of her memory loss. I realized how paranoid and scary this situation must be for Grace. It was overwhelming to me that simple memories were lost to her. As we drove through Ohio and saw animals in fields, Grace asked, "What were those things?"

One time I replied, "They are horses."

Grace quickly asked, "What are horses?"

I patiently described a horse and said that horses could be ridden or used to pull things.

Grace stared out into the passing fields, bewildered.

In another few miles, Grace asked, "What are those?"

"They are cows," I responded

Grace quickly asked, "What are cows?"

I patiently described a cow and said that the milk we drink comes from cows.

Grace continued to stare out the window at the passing scenes, which were all new to her in her mind.

Stopping at a rest area, the unfamiliarity with the facilities was another example of memories lost. I became concerned for Grace's safety during this journey, let alone this car trip. Quickly, I tried to reteach as much as I could as quickly as I could to protect her and keep her safe.

As we approached the end of our long drive, we faced introducing Grace to her dear grandparents and her loving brother.

It would take courage to say, "These are your grandparents" or "This is Michael, your brother." I prayed for strength and courage to face the ultimate awkward situation, with God's gracious help and His arms wrapped around me.

The sadness in each introduction was fourfold: mine, Frank's, Grace's, and the person she was meeting. We each had to have our own strength.

"Dear Lord, what could be sadder or harder?" I asked.

My parents met us at the door as we drove up to the house we had rented with them.

"Grace, this is O"—this was the name by which she had always known her grandmother. "She is your grandmother." Tears welled up in my eyes, my husband's eyes, and in my mother's and father's eyes. This was heartbreaking.

"Lord, please hold onto us," I prayed.

"Hi," Grace said shyly and gave her grandmother a hug.

"And this is Pops, your grandfather." I could barely speak by this point as the emotions rose.

Grace quietly gave her grandfather a hug and tried to smile.

My parents looked to me with puzzled glances, seeming to wonder if Grace remembered them now. I quietly shook my head and told them we would talk a little later.

"What are you going to do?" my dad asked.

That was a difficult question. All I knew to do was pray and stay focused on the human aspect of this illness, which meant making appointments and teaching Grace as much as she could tolerate each day.

Grace's grandparents were overwhelmed with emotion and found it hard to talk. They wanted answers and were anxious to get the problem "fixed." These were the same feelings my husband and I had been experiencing for two weeks already. A quick "fix" was not becoming apparent, as there was not a diagnosis and therefore no treatment plan.

Rather than focusing on the bewilderment and emptiness after the introductions to Grace's grandparents, I began to show Grace around the house, which had been familiar to her just three short weeks ago when we were last here.

Within fifteen minutes, the front door opened, and Michael, our son, walked in with his huge smile. I was so excited and overwhelmed to see him. Yet I carefully and prayerfully introduced him to Grace. "This is your brother, Michael."

Grace had the same response as when she was introduced to her grandparents; she said "Hi" with a hug.

After hugs and tears and smiles of joy, I continued to teach and teach and teach. Within a few hours, after a very long drive, it was time for bed. I sat with Grace as she told me, "I don't remember them at all, Mom." She had hoped seeing them would help her to remember them. No connections were made.

I told her, "You will get to know them as best as you can." I reassured her that they loved her in special ways, and she was safe to be with them.

During this trip, Grace and I discussed the possibilities we were facing with this journey of memory loss and severe headaches. We talked a lot about school.

With tears, Grace begged me, "Mom, promise me that you will never send me back to school." Grace was aware of what she did not know. She knew this was socially awkward, and she feared returning to middle school. There was enough cognitive awareness to know that much. Yet she did not know numbers, the alphabet, people in her life, or memories of special occasions.

As we lay there on the bed that evening, tearfully I said, "I promise you never have to return to school if you do not want to go." I promised Grace we would pursue other educational options for her. I processed many thoughts about abuse and threats that might have indeed caused this sudden onset of memory loss for Grace. I would remain her mother, protector, advocate, and nurse forever. This was my promise to Grace in the name of our Lord.

We spent three days visiting, and then it was time to say good-bye and return home for our work obligations. We would not send Grace to school, but we would continue to pursue treatment options for her headaches and diagnostic work-ups for the reason for her memory loss. The school district's policy was to start homebound instruction after the student missed forty consecutive days of school due to illness. We still had several weeks to wait until homebound instruction would officially begin through the school district.

Grace's grandmother felt she could not be away from the situation any longer. She returned home with us to be a support during the journey, while Grace's grandfather stayed to support our son at boarding school. Distance during a crisis is difficult. We would "divide and conquer" the situations that God had provided us. We would get through these situations as a family and with renewed strength and faith.

Having Grace's grandmother at home would be an advantage. She would be Grace's alternative care provider, so that I could continue teaching as a profession, part-time. In addition, she would be the additional psychosocial support to help with the many stressors of the journey. She would be the creator of projects and recipes to try during the lengthy days ahead. She would be the extra set of hands to rake leaves and shovel snow with Grace. She would be the extra set of eyes and ears to help endure the lengthy rides and the lengthy physician appointments of our journey.

A year earlier, our family life had changed by our son's attending a boarding school seven hundred miles away. He was an ice hockey goal tender, and his coaches wanted him to have the opportunity to play on a team with college scouts. This would be a way for him to play collegiate ice hockey, which was one of his dreams. The song lyrics "I'm letting go of the life I planned for me" by Francesca Battistelli became a praise song I listened to frequently.

I had always been a very involved mother of two, while working twenty to twenty-four hours per week and being involved in community activities. Yet I craved time alone. If I planned to have a day off by myself and then something changed, I would be extremely disappointed. Our society message of "me time" had been heard millions of times. As we sent my son off the first year, "letting go of the life I planned for me" was a wonderful message.

Now, one year later, I really had to let go of the life I planned for me. This was a personal wake-up call from God to me. We each have gifts that God wants us to use in our lives. Grace's illness made me realize my gift was being with others. I was not meant to be alone. I can't do God's work sufficiently when I am alone. Since the first weeks of Grace's illness, I had never felt the resentment that I used to feel when my "alone time" was changed by life's circumstances. I experienced an intense epiphany of God's hands and plans in my life.

Also, during the first weeks of Grace's illness, I realized and discussed with my friends and families that we were on a "journey." I knew this was a journey God had given to us for a reason. Truly, not understanding the reason at the time did not bother me.

Daily, I said, "This is a journey, but we do not know how long the journey will be."

We continued on the journey and did our best to make each day the brightest that it could be. This provided an overall calming feeling on daily life. Moments of anxiety would arise, but overall, we were calm and bright. Happiness prevailed during most of our days.

OCTOBER 20-31, 2009

You intended to harm me, but God intended it for good to accomplish what is now being done, the saving of many lives.—Genesis 50:20 NIV

We returned home from our weekend trip to visit with Grace's brother and grandparents to complete Grace's diagnostic testing. Once each diagnostic test was completed, we anxiously waited for the results from the physicians. We continued to pray for guidance as we waited for a diagnosis. We felt with certainty that there was a physical reason for Grace's sudden memory loss and severe headaches.

As Grace moved through each day as a new beginning and learning as much as she could tolerate for the day, I realized how very fortunate we were. Grace was able to remember everything she learned each consecutive day. She was content with being home, and she felt safe. When she wasn't in pain and during the few hours a day that she felt good, she was happy to participate in low-stress activities. I began to ponder her safety. She was fourteen years old and had been developmentally age appropriate before becoming severely ill. Maintaining her age-specific developmental level became an important focus, within the limits given in this situation.

However, I was concerned about her basic safety. *What if Grace went outside and wandered away from the house?* I thought. She did not know which house was ours, even though we had lived in this neighborhood for seven years. I retaught her which house was ours and even quizzed her on the matter as we drove into the neighborhood frequently. She relearned which people lived in the houses around us, but I was concerned that she might not remember in an emergency.

Yet what if she did go outside and didn't know her way back home? She physically appeared normal. Would the neighbors even know that she needed help getting home? We had a neighborhood directory, an e-mail list. I notified the neighbors of Grace's condition and asked them to please help her if they should find her wandering around in the neighborhood. Through God's love, my fears never materialized, and He kept Grace safe and close to her physical home.

In the meantime, unfortunately, the EEG and the MRI did not lead to a physical abnormality for Grace's sudden long-term memory loss and severe headaches. This was becoming a bigger and bigger mystery each day of our journey. Now we were left in the hands of the psychiatrist to establish a treatment plan for our daughter.

"What could have happened to our normal teenage daughter to manifest total long-term memory loss?" I repeatedly asked myself, day and night. I was filled with sadness as we anticipated treatment to help her to feel better, hopefully soon.

Two more appointments with the psychiatrist and further diagnostic testing still did not identify physical abnormalities. With no physical evidence for Grace's long-term memory loss and severe headaches, the psychiatrist diagnosed Grace with a conversion disorder. As a final step in the process of diagnosis, the psychiatrist attempted to hypnotize Grace. His theory was that Grace would easily be hypnotized if she truly had a conversion disorder.

My husband and I left the meeting room during the hypnosis. After fifteen minutes, the psychiatrist asked us to return to the meeting room and asked Grace to sit in the reception area while he had a discussion with us.

The psychiatrist said he had been unable to hypnotize Grace during the session. He was puzzled, as he had been confident he would hypnotize Grace and diagnose her with a conversion disorder. This meant yet another dead end—no diagnosis; no treatment plan.

Questions began racing through my mind. *Is this good news or bad news? What's the next step?*

The psychiatrist told us, "Grace has too many positive gains from staying home from school for two weeks."

"What do you mean by that?" I asked.

He listed as positive gains certain situations that we had described to him. "She has too many fun things going on at home. She can sleep as much as she wants. She doesn't have to do school work. And she can eat whatever she wants." Then, he boldly stated with authority, "Grace needs to get back to school and into a normal routine to facilitate her recovery."

Our appointment ended. That was the recommendation. That was the prescribed treatment plan. "Send her back to school" so she can face reality.

We quietly got in the car for the drive home. Grace immediately asked, "What did he say to you?"

"He said you should go back to school," I answered, shaking and in tears.

"But Mom, you promised me I don't ever have to go back to school," Grace quietly stated.

I tried to console Grace to the best of my ability. "I know, honey. You don't have to go back to school. We don't have to do what the doctor says." I continued, "Dad and I will decide what is best for you."

We had been anxiously waiting to establish a treatment plan for Grace. Now, the psychiatrist's only recommendation was that Grace should not be allowed to stay home any longer, because the sooner she got back to school, the better she would handle this.

Less than three weeks into this journey, I continued pondering if the memory loss was from a traumatic assault; for example, bullying. If Grace's memory loss and severe headaches were from a traumatic assault, why would we send her back to "the lion's den"? At this point in the journey, we did not know that she hadn't been hurt by somebody or threatened—Grace could not recall the day before her memory loss.

"She needs to go back to school immediately" resounded in my mind.

I was vehemently opposed to the psychiatrist's recommendation. My heart pounded, and my entire body literally was trembling. I wanted to scream.

Frank, on the other hand, adamantly felt we should follow the psychiatrist's recommendation to send Grace to school. He believed the doctor knew best.

I cried out, "Why would we do that?"

"The doctor says that would be best," Frank reiterated.

As a nurse for twenty-five years, I have provided care for many patients who will agree with whatever the doctor says. These patients view the physicians as God in some ways.

Unbelievable, I think again. This situation was showing me so many unbelievable moments. This was similar to the neurology team at the Children's Hospital recommending psychiatric treatment for Grace as an in-patient, with which I had not agreed. These were God's messages to keep me focused on being persistent in finding the best treatment for Grace.

I had promised Grace that I would not send her back to school until she felt well enough.

I continued to process thoughts about what might have happened that Grace did not want to go back to school. After promising that she did not have to go back to school, I continued by saying, "I can homeschool you if necessary."

Even though a medical professional's treatment plan included her going to school, I had promised her that wouldn't happen. In addition, Grace was in the ninth grade. She wouldn't know anybody. She wouldn't know anything about her school. She couldn't count past three. She didn't know the alphabet. *How could she be expected to go to school?* I pondered. *She would be eaten alive.*

I stood firm on my opinions—disagreeing with my husband and the psychiatrist—and refused to send Grace to school while she suffered severe headaches and total memory loss.

Little did I know that this would be the first time I would become so profoundly aware of my resilient character—in this situation and other life situations. I simply would not accept an answer that seemed so far-fetched. I would not allow others to control my daughter's destiny. I would not give up until we had some definitive answers. Professionals would give us information that did not make sense. Sometimes these were bumps in the road; sometimes these were roadblocks. But I never gave up. I relied on my family and friends for inner strength to continue the daily battles and to listen and hear what I was thinking. I relied on my resources and my professionalism to manage our journey to the best of my ability. We continued to pray for guidance and patience during the journey, but God was not providing us with any direct answers yet.

A bright spot in one of Grace's days was during October. One of my friends came to "kid-sit" and brought a pumpkin. My friend said, "We are going to carve it, if Grace is up to it."

"Right now, Grace doesn't know what a pumpkin is or a jack-o-lantern," I informed my friend. This was an opportunity for my friend to reteach Grace. To me, this was how every day proceeded—by realizing Grace didn't remember certain things and reteaching her. I came home that day from work to a jack-o-lantern and roasted pumpkin seeds. I smiled and listened to my friend tell me about the time she had spent with Grace.

Angela was our prayer warrior. Repeatedly, one thing kept coming to Angela in her prayers: Grace had been diagnosed with Lyme disease two months prior to the onset of memory loss and severe headaches.

Lyme disease was identified in 1974 when researchers investigated an unusually large number of juvenile rheumatoid arthritis in Lyme, Connecticut. The children affected had a peculiar skin rash before they developed arthritis symptoms, which was unusual. Lyme disease is caused by the *Borrelia burgdorferi* bacteria. Deer ticks carry this organism and transmit the disease to other animals or humans. When humans are infected with Lyme disease, they may observe "bull's-eye"-type rashes on their bodies. However, the bull's-eye does not always appear in every person infected. If a person does not see the deer tick or does not have a bull's-eye rash, the diagnosis of Lyme disease will often not be made. A person may experience flu-like symptoms, including body aches, low-grade fever, stiff neck, swollen lymph nodes, headaches, fatigue, muscle aches, and joint pain. These symptoms could become persistent when infected with Lyme disease, rather than improving, as when experiencing the flu. After being infected with Lyme disease for longer periods without treatment, other symptoms may develop. These symptoms may include arthritis, stiff neck, severe headaches, numbness and weakness of the extremities, memory loss, difficulty concentrating, and changes in mood. The documented memory loss with Lyme disease has been short-term memory loss, such as forgetting where you put the car keys or and forgetting to run an errand.

We had included the information about Grace's diagnosis of Lyme disease in our discussion with each treating physician. None of the health-care professionals we encountered had made a connection between Lyme disease and this sudden onset of long-term memory loss and severe headaches. Angela, however, had been led through prayer to realize Grace's prior diagnosis was important in getting a diagnosis and treatment plan. Upon reviewing the literature, I found short-term memory loss was well documented with Lyme disease but not long-term memory loss. Quite frankly, each physician treating Grace stated this long-term memory loss and severe headaches could *not* be related to Lyme disease.

NOVEMBER 1-14, 2009

When Jesus spoke again to the people, he said, "I am the light of the world. Whoever follows me will never walk in darkness, but will have the light of life."—John 8:12 NIV

Throughout the month of diagnostic testing and appointments, I continued discussing with Angela the possibility of Lyme disease involvement.

"You've told each of the doctors about her Lyme disease, and they haven't done anything with that information," Angela told me.

Angela was right. But where did we go from here? Angela had the name of a Lyme-literate specialist, which she gave to me.

By this point in our journey, the physicians had not found any physical abnormality causing Grace's sudden long-term memory loss. The EEG and the MRI were inconclusive, meaning the results were normal. I made a phone call to Mary, the Lyme-literate specialist, and scheduled an appointment. Mary could see Grace within the next four days. Praise be to God.

We definitely needed to get some answers. Grace continued to suffer severe, incapacitating headaches, with light and noise sensitivity. She couldn't leave the house for more than a quick errand. She couldn't watch television. She didn't know what an iPod was for. She didn't know what a cell phone was. She didn't know what a computer was or what it was used for.

"What do you do with these?" was a question that echoed throughout each day.

Through Angela's loving advice, one month into this journey we had the first appointment with a Lyme-literate specialist. As we entered the reception area of Mary's office, we were handed a questionnaire to complete about symptoms that Grace may have experienced. The question I most recall was "Have you been told this is all in your head?" Bingo. This sounded like we were on the right track.

Mary was a physician's assistant who personally suffered from infection with Lyme disease. She spent ninety minutes with Grace for this appointment. The first portion of the appointment was spent on Grace's history, followed by a thorough assessment.

Mary discussed the diagnostic portion of Lyme disease. She described the blood work that would confirm Grace's likely infection with Lyme disease. A paramount element in successful treatment of Lyme disease was an accurate diagnosis of Lyme disease and its potential co-infections. However, diagnosing Lyme disease accurately was not an easy task. First, the symptoms often are vague and mimic other illnesses and infections. Second, the most commonly used diagnostic screening tests for Lyme disease often yield inaccurate results. Up to one-third of Lyme disease cases have been misdiagnosed due to a high rate of "false negative" results. A "false negative" result means the laboratory results indicate the person is negative for the organism when the person does in fact have active Lyme disease.[1]

Mary described to us the additional challenges in diagnosing Lyme disease. If a person has removed a tick from his skin and has a classic bull's-eye rash at the tick-bite site, then the diagnosis is less complicated. However, the deer tick is very small—as small as the period at the end of this sentence. Glance at the cover of this book. The small "speck" in the glow of the candle is the size of a deer tick. Prompt and accurate removal of a deer tick would prevent the transmission of Lyme disease, but the tick is very difficult to find on an animal or human body. Not everyone will develop the characteristic rash, and the symptoms that a person does have may be nonspecific and flu-like in the early stages, with joint pain that develops into chronic arthritis and/or neurological symptoms that appear months later.

In addition, Grace would be tested for other tick-borne diseases as well as opportunistic infections. These infections were possible, as Lyme disease likely had weakened Grace's immune system.

---

[1]   www.LymeDisease.org/lyme101/lyme_disease/lyme_diagnosis.html.

This appointment was psychologically overwhelming to me. I sat there and absorbed as many details as I could. It was only Mary, Grace, and me in the examination room. I had not brought any family or friends with me to this appointment. This was the one appointment along this journey for which I do not recall the actual conversation or the questions asked.

Mary recommended homeopathic treatments along with antibiotics, which were started immediately. Lab work was sent to the *only* laboratory in the United States that specializes in tick-borne diseases.

Mary inundated us with information on what to expect as treatment began for Grace's infections. Grace would likely endure *Herxheimer reaction* as the antibiotic treatment began. The Herxheimer reaction was believed to be an immunological reaction caused by the bacteria dying. As the antibiotic attacked the bacteria, the bacteria would release a substance into the blood faster than the body could get rid of them. Mary stated the symptoms Grace was suffering would likely get worse for up to two weeks after the medications were started. These symptoms might include increased joint and muscle pain, increased headaches or fatigue, chills and fever, low blood pressure, and increased heart rate.

Mary outlined a plan to manage the Herxheimer reaction. Grace's diet should be more natural, with fewer processed foods, more green vegetables, less sugar, and gluten-free. These changes in Grace's diet would decrease the ability for the bacteria to survive. Another measure would be to take baths with Epsom salts or hydrogen peroxide. As the specialist explained, we were using the body's largest organ, the skin, to draw out the dying bacteria.

In anticipation of the diagnosis, Mary provided me with a list of Lyme-literate physicians to contact. As a physician's assistant, Mary could not order the intravenous antibiotics that Grace would likely need. She recommended making an appointment with a Lyme-literate physician to prescribe intravenous antibiotics. She warned me that the Lyme-literate physicians would likely have a three- to six-month waiting list.

Mary provided us with a list of "Lyme disease rules" to follow during the treatment to improve Grace's symptoms and to facilitate her treatment. Fatigue was a major symptom of Lyme disease, and getting enough rest was very important to the treatment plan. A diet with high-quality protein and fiber that was low in fat and low in carbohydrates was recommended. There is nothing quick about healing from Lyme disease. "Patient endurance produces godliness" was listed on the Lyme disease rules.

Mary also recommended dietary guidelines to support the treatment regimen. Lyme disease was caused by *spirochetes* (a type of bacteria) in the blood. These organisms needed to live off of something, and they thrived on sugar. Therefore, the recommended dietary guidelines included foods with a low glycemic index, that were gluten-free and yeast-free, and that were not fermented. Recommended foods included fresh fruits and vegetables and meats.

The morning after this first appointment with Mary, I called each Lyme-literate physician provided on the list and tried to make an appointment with each one taking new patients. The earliest any of the physicians would be able to schedule an appointment to see Grace was in two months. I asked each of the offices to place Grace on the cancellation list. If they had a cancellation, they would call us to get Grace in sooner.

I prepared the suggested foods and encouraged Grace to eat small amounts every two hours to keep her nutritional status stable within the guidelines provided. She would eat the portion given to her and not desire extra food at all. At one point Grace said, "I would die if I was alone and nobody fed me."

Each day was filled with prayers. I asked God for answers and for continued patience through this journey. Mary had told us the results would be available in a week.

A week after the appointment, as I was driving home from work, my husband called me and told me to call the Lyme-literate specialist immediately. Frank said Mary's message was that the laboratory results were in and to call her back immediately. As I drove, I calmly called and spoke directly with Mary. The news was grim but not unexpected. Not only was Grace infected with Lyme disease, but she was also infected with five other organisms. Two other primary infections were babeiosis and mycoplasma infection. Lyme disease and babeiosis are borne diseases, carried and transmitted by the deer tick.

Organisms causing co-infections could be transmitted to a person at the same time that Lyme disease is transmitted, or the organisms may infect the person at a different time. A major co-infection to Lyme disease is babeiosis, caused by *Babesia microti*, a parasitic organism. The deer tick also carries the organism and transmits the disease to other animals or humans. When a human is infected with babeiosis, symptoms may include fever, chills, sweats, and fatigue. In addition, humans may develop hemolytic anemia, jaundice, headaches, myalgia (muscle pain), arthralgia (joint pain), or anorexia.[2]

Current literature on babeiosis disease indicated that 20 percent of those infected die from the infection. This was in the immune-compromised population, primarily the elderly and very young. Babeiosis was the number-one infectious blood-transmitted illness in the United States. The northeastern states have begun testing donated blood to prevent transmission of the disease through the blood supply. The Federal Drug Administration (FDA) acknowledged the significance of this infection, because it can now be transmitted through the nation's blood supply. Perhaps the medical community and the insurance companies will follow in the treatment protocols and help to diagnose and treat this deadly disease. Statistics from the Centers for Disease Control indicated there were nearly three times as many confirmed cases of Lyme disease in our county, Bucks County, from 1992 to 2011.[3]

"Grace is really sick," Mary quietly told me. She said Grace had to be seen by a Lyme-literate specialist physician as soon as possible to get intravenous antibiotics started.

Where in the world is this journey going? I asked God. *How will we get through this?* With God's help and mercy, we continued on the journey faithfully.

Mary had told us that Lyme disease and the co-infections were treatable once diagnosed. Antibiotics would be prescribed to kill the organisms. Current medical protocol for treatment of newly diagnosed, non-complicated Lyme disease was an antibiotic for two to four weeks, yet Mary recommended six weeks. Controversy raged between the

---

[2]   www.LymeDisease.org/lyme101/lyme_disease/lyme_symptoms.html

[3]   http://www.cdc.gov/lyme/stats

general medical professions and the specialists. The medical insurance companies' reimbursement and coverage was based on the standard medical protocols.

Now, Mary was telling us that Grace's illness was in advanced stages and would need intensive antibiotic therapy, along with holistic treatment. Grace would need much more than the prescribed oral antibiotic for two to four weeks.

We would have to wait for the Lyme-literate physician appointment. In the meantime, we continued the prescribed oral antibiotics from Mary. We continued to implement the Lyme disease rules and the other homeopathic methods prescribed.

Within a week, when I got home from work, Grace told me, "Dr. L's office called. They have an appointment tomorrow at one. I told them we could make it to that appointment."

"What?" I was confused.

"Dr. L is the Lyme doctor, Mom," Grace explained.

"Wait a minute. She can see you tomorrow?"

"Yes. I told her we would call her back if we can't make it." Grace was clear on the details.

"This is amazing." I grabbed my pile of papers on the dining room table. This appointment was not meant to happen for weeks. God had answered our prayers. Grace would be seen by a Lyme-literate physician much sooner than expected. Praise be to God.

The following morning, we woke up early. I was excited, as if I was going on a trip. My mother rode with us to Dr. L's office, a nearly two-hour drive from our home. The appointment was for one o'clock. As we drove, Grace moaned most of the way. She continued to have severe headaches and light sensitivity. It was a bright, sunny fall day. We encouraged her to cover her head with the blanket as much as possible, since she was sensitive to the bright light and sunshine. We encouraged her to snack on small amounts of food. We prayed and hoped for relief and further answers from Dr. L.

Upon arriving at Dr. L's office we completed the required paperwork and sat in the waiting room. The wait seemed to go on forever. We waited for two hours before Dr. L saw us. We complained to each other that this was an unacceptable amount of time to wait for a scheduled appointment. We tried to pass the time by looking at magazines and chatting. Grace was more and more miserable throughout the uncomfortable wait. We had driven two hours and now had waited two hours. This would literally take us all day.

We were blessed to finally meet Dr. L but admittedly irritated by then. I asked God for patience in this grueling situation. We needed this doctor, no matter how much we didn't like the way the office was managed. Dr. L reviewed the laboratory findings and assessment Mary had forwarded. Dr. L reiterated the details of the infectious diseases in Grace's body. She reviewed the Lyme disease rules with us. Dr. L suffered with Lyme disease and was on a mission to help others fight these infections. She said, "It will take faith, family, and friends to survive this disease."

Dr. L recommended further supplements to help rid the organisms from Grace's body. She reminded us of the Herxheimer reaction and the intensity of Grace's symptoms as they worsened before any improvement would be possible. We scheduled an appointment for the insertion of the intravenous line for the following Tuesday, in five days. The intravenous line would be started in Dr. L's office by a certified registered nurse. In the meantime, we would coordinate obtaining the IV antibiotics, arrange for a visiting IV nurse for weekly lab work and IV dressing changes, and ask for insurance authorization to pay for the medication for a month.

I told Dr. L we had an appointment with the pediatric hospital neurologist for the next day.

"You are not going there," Dr. L stated.

"But this is an appointment for Grace's headaches and memory loss," I feebly stated.

"You are done with the mainstream medical model. They will not help you," Dr L continued.

I was aghast. *What? Cancel the appointment with the neurologist?* I thought. *Is this the right thing to do?* I prayed for guidance. I was scared.

By five o'clock in the afternoon, we got in the car to drive home. Unbelievable—we had been blessed for Grace to be seen by Dr. L, but we were exhausted. Now, we needed to drive home. As I drove, we ate the lunch we had packed and chatted quietly.

Once Grace was being treated by the specialist, we were told we were "outside of traditional medicine." As a nurse, this made me personally a little cautious and apprehensive.

The following week, we prepared for another long trip to Dr. L's office for the insertion of Grace's intravenous line. The ride was a little more bearable, knowing where we were going and the amount of waiting we would endure. Again, my mother rode with us for moral support and diversion during the long hours ahead.

Upon arrival at Dr. L's office, we were in an exam room within half an hour—thankfully. We weren't seeing Dr. L, so we moved through the office quicker. The nurse who would insert the intravenous line arrived and prepared Grace. Within half an hour, the IV line was in, and we were leaving the office.

The insurance company had approved thirty days of IV antibiotics for Grace. The medication and supplies would arrive the following day. An infusion therapy nurse would make a home visit the next day to change the IV dressing. This was a big step in beginning the treatment for the infections in Grace's body.

The days were long and difficult. Along with the medical aspect of Grace's illness, one month into the journey the school district began sending homebound instructors to our home to cover the four academic courses for ninth grade. At first, the instructors did not know where to start. I had retaught Grace her numbers, math facts, and simple math. Grace had retained the ability to read. English, science, and social studies, therefore, could continue on the current topics being covered in school. These were not cumulative topics and therefore were easier to master. Math, on the other hand, is a cumulative subject, and Grace needed to be retaught everything before beginning with Algebra II.

I continued to update our friends and family through frequent, often daily, e-mails. One friend offered to set up a blog for me to communicate, but I wasn't sure how public I wanted this journey to be on the Internet. I opted to communicate through e-mails instead. Friends and families asked for ways that they could help. I already had many of them "kid-sitting," bringing an occasional meal, or running errands. Now, with Grace's intravenous line, she was self-conscious about people seeing her IV. So I asked that when my friends were out shopping that they purchase cute knee-high socks, maybe even to go with the different holidays. I would cut out the feet of these socks and use them as a sleeve for Grace's arm, to cover up her intravenous line. This gave our friends a way to participate and to help and a fun way for Grace to cover her IV. God had again provided for us through His graciousness.

NOVEMBER 23, 2009

O Lord my God, I called to you for help
And you healed me.
O Lord, you brought me up from the grave
You spared me from going down into the pit.—*Psalm 30:2-3 NIV*

Less than two months into our journey, Grace had a major life-threatening complication. The day before Thanksgiving, the infusion nurse, Terri, visited our home to assess and change the dressing on Grace's IV. Grace was sitting at the dining room table when Terri arrived, so Terri agreed to do her assessment and Grace's IV dressing change in the dining room, as Grace was already there and comfortable. After completing her assessment, Terri began to remove the old dressing from Grace's IV. Within a few seconds, Grace became pale and nonresponsive. Her eyes glazed over as she stared off into the distance. Next, Grace fainted and slumped over in the chair.

Terri directed me to help lift Grace from the chair and lay her down with her feet elevated. This would allow the blood to get to Grace's brain. Unfortunately, in her debilitated condition, Grace's body did not react as it would have with a "normal" fainting spell.

I screamed up the stairs for my son to come to the dining room quickly. My parents had driven Michael home from boarding school for Thanksgiving. He had arrived home less than an hour earlier. As he came into the dining room, I quickly told him, "Grace has fainted." Michael helped Terri and me to reposition Grace across three chairs at the dining room table. This would allow blood to flow to Grace's brain and hopefully restore her level of consciousness.

Terri continued to take Grace's blood pressure and pulse.

Grace would be alert for about ten seconds and then pass out again.

"She needs to get to the hospital!" I frantically said to Terri.

"Give her a few minutes," Terri responded. "She will come out of it."

Michael called my parents to tell them of Grace's deteriorating condition and that they should go to the hospital to meet me there.

I was panicking. "I'll call for the ambulance."

"No, she is going to be okay," Terri insisted. "Plus, you would be better off to drive her to the hospital on your own. By the time the ambulance gets here, you could have her there. They can't really do anything for her during the transport anyway."

Grace opened her eyes for a few seconds, and we tried to get her to drink some juice. As soon as she swallowed the juice, she lost consciousness again.

Grace's pulse was low, and her blood pressure was low.

I repeated, "I think I better call for the ambulance."

Terri again stated, "It would be best for you to transport her." I asked Michael to drive the car up to the front door so we could carry Grace into the car.

The following was a surreal experience and still seems so, even as I recall the details about this part of our journey. Michael carried Grace to the car and put her in the front seat, reclining it as far as it would go. I got in the driver's seat and began driving across the yard into the street and toward the hospital.

I was terrified, unlike any other time in my life. I was praying out loud and talking to Grace in a loud voice. We were in God's hands, being transported to the hospital. Without God at that moment, Grace would have died in the car. She lapsed in and out of consciousness continually during that fifteen-minute drive. I knew she was dying, and only God could get us there.

As I drove, Grace's fingertips turned blue.

Her fingernails were blue.

She did not have oxygen circulating to her fingers.

She did not have oxygen circulating to her brain.

As she came to, I would tell her, "Clap your hands and stomp your feet." My thought was that Grace's moving would at least keep her blood circulating. "Please stay with me, Grace," I begged as I drove frantically across the country roads leading to the hospital. There were only three traffic lights and four stop signs along the way. I slowed down to make sure there was no traffic but kept on driving.

Tears poured from my eyes. I was gasping for each breath of my own. *How could this be happening?* "Dear Lord, what is happening to my girl?" I asked out loud. *"Why?"* simply kept coming out of my mouth. "Come on, Grace. Clap your hands. Stomp your feet," I demanded.

Her fingertips were blue.

Her fingernails were blue.

She did not have oxygen circulating to her fingers.

She did not have oxygen circulating to her brain.

"Keep driving," God said.

Looking back at this situation, I made a very careless decision to personally transport Grace to the hospital, even though Terri insisted transporting Grace in our family car would be best. My resilience was low in this life-threatening moment, or I would have followed my knowledge and gotten an ambulance. But looking back, God was there, and He got Grace to the hospital.

Jesus said: "this sickness will not end in death. No, it is for God's glory so that God's Son may be glorified through it."—*John 11:4 NIV*

As I pulled up to the emergency room entrance, a stranger—a Good Samaritan—calmly walked by my car. He asked, "Do you need help?" He was a true Samaritan.

I frantically replied, with tears running down my cheeks, "Yes. This is my daughter. Can you help me get her into the emergency room, please?"

Without another word, he swiftly lifted Grace out of the car and put her in a wheelchair that was close by.

Then instantly, my mother came quickly walking toward us. I was so profoundly in God's hands that I couldn't say anything.

My mother wheeled Grace in through the door of the emergency room.

"There goes my girl," I sobbed as I hurriedly got in the car and went to park it in a nearby parking spot. I knew that Grace might be further into a crisis and could die before I could get to see her again.

I prayed and prayed with every breath that I took. I prayed for God's will to be done.

Then I ran into the triage area. Grace was not there. The nurse took one look at me and said, "They have taken your daughter back already into the emergency room." She came around from the desk and walked with me to the emergency room cubicle where they had taken Grace. My whole body was trembling.

This was the same hospital where Grace was initially seen with the sudden loss of long-term memory, seven weeks earlier.

Immediately, the treating emergency room physician came into the cubicle and said, "Did you ever treat her urinary tract infection from her last visit?"

"What? What infection?" I questioned.

"I remember your daughter from when she was here," the ER physician said. "I remember seeing her urinalysis from that visit showing bacteria. So you never got that treated?"

"No, we didn't," I abruptly responded.

The ER physician left the cubicle, and a nurse drew blood work and asked assessment information. "What's your name?

"Grace," my daughter responded.

"What's your birthday?" the nurse asked.

Grace stared at me. I began to update the nurse on the memory loss and severe headaches from which Grace had suffered during the past seven weeks. I thought, *Here we go again, having to explain everything.*

What was going on here? The urinary tract infection hadn't been treated. Thinking back, Grace's pediatrician had called to follow up from her initial emergency room visit. During that conversation, he mentioned the lab work indicated bacteria in her urine. The pediatrician specifically had asked me seven weeks ago, "Is Grace having discomfort when urinating?"

I had asked Grace, while on the phone with the pediatrician, if it hurt when she peed, and she said it was fine.

The pediatrician had said, "That is the only abnormal lab. I'm sure it couldn't be causing her memory loss. Since she is asymptomatic, we are not going to treat it."

Oh Lord, now I started to think she had a urinary tract infection that had become septic and spread throughout her body. This could have been prevented if it had been treated. How could such an infection not be treated?

My mind was racing while my body continued to tremble. These fainting spells could be a result of this infection spreading through her body as well as the other diagnoses, which she was receiving intravenous medications to treat. Why hadn't she received a prescription to treat this urinary tract infection at the onset of her memory loss, seven weeks earlier? I continued to process overwhelming amounts of information as Grace's mother and as a nurse.

Months later, after the infection was treated, we put the pieces together and realized that Grace wasn't able to notice the burning when she urinated because she did not remember what it felt like to urinate without discomfort.

Several nurses continued to assess and work around Grace's bedside in the emergency room cubicle. Grace continued to lapse into unconsciousness throughout the first hour in the ER. The ER physician ordered IV fluids to stabilize Grace, but during Grace's initial collapse at home, her intravenous line got pulled out of her arm. She needed a new intravenous access.

I explained to Grace, "The IV nurse will be putting in another IV for you."

Grace's face was full of fear. This was unlike Grace. She had always been a person to be brave.

I held Grace's hand tightly and reassured her to the best of my ability. "You need the IV to get better. It won't take long."

The infusion nurse, Meredith, came into the ER cubicle to insert a new long-term intravenous line. The intravenous line needed to be inserted under sterile conditions, so she asked me to leave the cubicle.

I understood the premise of the sterile field, but this was my young daughter. Ethically, I felt I should be allowed to stay at least in the corner of the cubicle. A child should not have to be alone at a time of such high stress and fear.

I sheepishly walked from the cubicle. I stood firmly right outside the glass door and peeked in through the gap in the opening of the privacy curtain. Grace could see me. And I could see her. Meredith was obviously having a difficult time with the insertion of the intravenous line. She stoically continued with her work, not saying a word to Grace. Meredith took one intravenous catheter out and started the procedure over again.

I was humbled like never before. I cried and prayed. This was the closest Grace had come to dying during this journey. I saw tears in Grace's eyes, and her nose turned red as she cried away her fears during this procedure. Prayers flowed continuously over Grace and the situation. "God, this is a wonderful Christian servant; a little girl with a huge heart who reaches out to those in need. This is the girl who makes friends out of the underdogs in the world. Please give her the chance to continue your work here on earth. Let God's will be done, whatever that may be."

After four attempts, the new intravenous line was in. Meredith left the cubicle without a word. Without a smile. Without a thoughtful gesture.

I could hardly contain myself as I rushed to Grace's bedside, and we hugged and cried together until the ER nurse came in to start IV fluids. Grace received an antibiotic to begin the treatment for the urinary tract infection.

Within several hours, we were on our way home from this emergency room visit.

Now, we had a new diagnosis that was treatable with an antibiotic and a new intravenous line—and many more questions:

Where are we headed?

Will she have further fainting spells?

If so, where will she be when they happen?

Will she be stable enough to get to the emergency room?

As if living with a teenage daughter who had lost her memory wasn't a challenge enough, now we had more issues.

Apprehension abounded as I wondered what would happen next. It literally took all of my strength to get through each moment. Who could answer these questions for me? No one had been on this journey before. None of the physicians knew what to expect. None of the physicians could give me expected outcomes. I relied on God to fulfill and sustain me.

The following morning, Grace received a bouquet of balloons from one of our friends. Grace said, "I really felt bad yesterday, and today Joy sent these balloons." Grace smiled the biggest smile. Those balloons lasted for a month. I put them around the house to spread the joy. God had provided us with the love and support of friends to help us through the toughest times.

Grace continued receiving infusions of the prescribed intravenous antibiotics each day at home—this, along with sixteen pills each day. As my son noted on his visit home, "It looks like she is an old woman with all of these medications." True. This was a different lifestyle. This was necessary to keep her alive during this journey. Even with taking all of these medications, there were no definitive answers or expectations of recovery. This was the reality of many people living with a chronic or terminal illness. Humans endure a tremendous amount to save their own lives or the lives of their loved ones.

Although an infusion nurse visited once a week to change the IV dressing and to draw blood, I, as Grace's caregiver, cared for the intravenous line every day and infused the prescribed antibiotics. Fortunately, this was something I had performed hundreds, if not thousands, of times as a nurse. I quickly realized the psychological aspect of caring for my daughter would impact my ability to perform ordinary nursing skills. I could barely control my apprehension each day. Never did I believe I would be apprehensive about infusing an antibiotic. Infusing fluids and medications were skills that nurses used several times every day at work in hospitals. For each of Grace's infusions, I prayed for the strength to administer the medication and to see tomorrow in a fresh way.

The Lyme-literate specialist had discussed the options of treatment. Intravenous antibiotics were the preferred treatment, but most health-care insurance companies did not cover the intravenous antibiotic used for Lyme disease. How could this be the situation?

I had often wondered how people managed to complete all of the daily management prescribed in a medical regimen at home. The prescribed medical regimen was in addition to everyday activities. In our society, we live hurried lives, and adding daily management of an illness to the scenario is a major stressor. Managing and coordinating Grace's care, along with appealing to the insurance company, became a full-time job.

DECEMBER 2009

Give us today our daily bread.—*Matthew 6:11 NIV*

Caring friends and family who visited while Grace was ill were welcomed. Grace was always cordial, even when she was in physical pain. She cherished her time with the visitors, but at this time in our journey, Grace did not recall any of these people from her past. She didn't remember the friends or what these friends had done with her in the past. I often wondered how she could reconnect with friends and families.

Grace spent many hours looking through her yearbooks and on Facebook, reacquainting herself with friends from school and activities. Yes, Facebook had great potential in helping somebody like Grace to reconnect.

Yet Grace was concerned about seeing her friends. She wondered what they thought was funny, what they talked about, and what they did together for fun.

Two of Grace's dear friends came and made a gingerbread house with Grace for a gingerbread competition before Christmas. The girls spent several hours on a few different days, making and decorating the house. Grace enjoyed being with them, but they were not familiar to her. When they left, Grace said, "I still don't remember them, Mom."

The greatest gift was having friends who were not afraid of the awkwardness of Grace's memory loss. God provided us with encouragement through these friends.

Early in December, Michelle, a friend at Bible study, had her birthday. We sang "Happy Birthday" and celebrated with a special lunch. When Grace and I got home from Bible study, Grace asked me, "Can you teach me that song?"

"What song, Grace?"

"The one we sang today for Michelle."

"You mean 'Happy Birthday'?" I realized Grace had not heard this song since before her memory loss.

I started singing, and after repeating the song several times, Grace was able to sing along with me. A precious memory returned to Grace through the grace of God.

We traveled every three to four weeks to see my son and father at the boarding school. We reintroduced airplane traveling to Grace. She loved being on the airplane, just like before losing her memory. She preferred traveling by plane, rather than by car. We had special dispensation for traveling through security with additional fluids, allowed for medical treatment. Security guards often questioned her about her intravenous line, which I believe was uncalled for, but in some sense, this questioning gave Grace recognition of her bravery and strength on this journey. Grace would say, "I'd rather have a broken leg because people can see that." Having memory loss is something others can't see. Memory loss is also something others do not understand. Unfortunately, even the health-care professionals do not understand memory loss.

Grace began enjoying our trips as a diversion to everyday life and routine. We would base our trips around appointments and her homebound instructor schedule.

During the visits with her grandfather, Grace relearned to play card games. She became known as a card shark, just as she was before her memory loss. She loved sitting and playing cards and winning the games. She readily laughed and enjoyed new experiences and rediscovery through these trips.

It was difficult to incorporate each of the components of the prescribed treatment regimen. Grace's treatment was not just taking the antibiotics. She was to rest as much as possible to allow her body to heal. The Lyme-literate specialist wanted Grace to use her skin to help excrete the spirochetes as they died. Grace would take a bath with hydrogen peroxide or Epsom salts in the water twice a day to facilitate this process. Her arm with the intravenous line had to stay dry, so I assisted Grace with bathing. One evening, I saw clumps of Grace's long hair in my hand as I washed her hair. This was too much; now Grace was going to lose her hair or have very thin hair? *"No, God, why?"* I asked quietly. The hair loss was a side effect of the antibiotics Grace was receiving.

One evening at home after dinner, Grace went into the living room where she often would sit and chat for most of the evening. Watching television in the family room wasn't of interest to her, and she couldn't tolerate the light or the noise for any length of time. This particular evening, as I cleaned up the dinner dishes, I heard Grace begin to play the piano in the living room. She sat at the piano and began to play a song she used to play. Grace had piano and instrument lessons throughout the years, but she never really was interested in playing any instruments. But here she was, playing a song on the piano when so many memories were gone. I said to Frank, "How can this be?" He looked at me with questioning eyes and disbelief. Grace quickly expressed an interest in learning how to read the music again and learning songs from the music books. This gave us a new task to teach Grace during our free time at home. She loved learning about music this time.

As Grace's fifteenth birthday approached, three months into the journey, she wanted to have a birthday party. In the past, we had simple birthday parties at our home versus big celebrations at party venues. I helped Grace to make the arrangements, and we invited eight girlfriends to our house. Only two of the girls had seen Grace since she had become ill.

We looked online at the grocery store bakery to pick out a cake. Grace chose a snowman cake made out of cupcakes. On an errand one day, we bought "Happy Birthday" paper plates and napkins. On the day of the party, we picked up the cake and a few balloons at the grocery store. This was a simple birthday celebration for our beautiful daughter.

The day of Grace's birthday party was beautiful with a recent snowfall. This was Grace's "first snow," as she didn't remember what snow was. This was a dream come true, as Grace had always wanted to have snow on her birthday. The girls took Grace out in the yard to go sledding. They loved sharing time with Grace, and she loved having them over. Again, each of them was not a familiar memory to Grace at this time.

The girlfriends sang "Happy Birthday" while Grace gave a guarded smile. She was in pain. Her head hurt, and she had been outside with the brightness of a snowy day. She was still sensitive to the light and loud sounds. Grace quietly opened the gifts the girls had brought for her birthday. We had planned for the party to be two hours, and that was appropriate for Grace's condition.

The girls each hugged Grace and said good-bye. The rest of the day was spent resting in the quiet, darkened family room.

Grace did not remember anything about trips and vacations we had taken in the past. Pictures allow us to visually connect our memories to the past, but showing pictures of our vacations to Grace did not help her to remember them. When I'd show Grace pictures from our past, I'd think, *Is it worth the emotional torment to delve into these albums? Does it benefit us in any way?*

A lesson to remember from this part of our journey is the importance of documenting life events. At some point, pictures may be a way to retrieve memories of the past for your loved one.

A friend came one day to kid-sit and brought her three-year-old son. They had come to stay with Grace several times before. During our conversation before I left for work, she told me that her son asked to pray for Grace each night during his bedtime prayers. Grace's life was touched and prayed for by friends and family of all ages from so many places. God was awesome to show us so much love through others.

The approaching holiday season would be Grace's "first Christmas." *Where do I begin to teach about Christmas?* I thought. *This is Jesus's birthday.* I quickly realized the amount of information and traditions related to Christmas that needed to be retaught to Grace. I wanted the holiday to be special and for Grace to rejoice in the birth of Jesus. Traditional holiday songs were not familiar to Grace. The season of Advent and the preparation for Christmas was not familiar to Grace. She did not recall decorations and traditional cooking. Grace enjoyed watching her dad put up the outside decorations: lights on the house one day and a Nativity scene on the lawn another day.

Grace's brother arrived home from boarding school a week before Christmas, and she enjoyed spending time with him. He was a little unsure of what Grace could and could not do. He also did not know what Grace had and had not relearned.

Imagine decorating a Christmas tree for the "first time." As a family, we went to the local tree farm and chose a fresh-cut Fraser Fir for our Christmas tree. Grace loved the smell of the tree. The day after getting the tree, we decorated it. We described the special ornaments to Grace, one by one. "This ornament is from our trip to Radio City Music Hall to see the Rockettes," I explained. Then this entailed explaining Radio City Music Hall in New York City and the Christmas show and the dancers, the Rockettes. Grace enjoyed relearning these moments, although she did not recall any additional information about the events and special occasions.

In the past, we had incorporated giving to the less fortunate into our Christmas. Through our church, we donated grocery-store gift cards, and we donated to Toys for Tots. Grace was able to relearn the joy of giving to others in the name of the Lord.

It was a very merry Christmas. We were blessed to celebrate the birth of Jesus. With caution, we proceeded through Christmas Day, which was tailored to meet the needs of Grace's treatment regimen. For example, the tradition of getting up at dawn to begin the celebration with opening presents was held later in the morning to provide enough rest for Grace. Another alteration in the tradition was a quieter, smaller dinner celebration for Christmas Day, with food that Grace was allowed to eat with her prescribed regimen. Everybody in the family tailored the day to meet Grace's needs. From the preparation for Christmas, to the Christmas Eve service, through the joy of Christmas Day, Grace's excitement and glee were exciting to witness.

At New Year's I spent time discussing this occasion with Grace—that we normally stayed at home and watched the ball drop in New York City's Time Square.

Our son was invited to spend the evening with some friends, so Grace and I drove him to his friend's home and then returned home. Frank was on a flight on New Year's Eve and New Year's Day. For New Year's Eve, Grace and I anticipated having a quiet evening at home, like many others since this journey began. However, Grace received a surprise phone call from Kathy, a friend she wouldn't have seen often under normal circumstances. Kathy wanted Grace to come over and "hang out" for the evening. Grace looked at me with happiness in her eyes. "Can I go?" she asked.

Grace had reacquainted herself with Kathy on Facebook during the past three months. Kathy was a lonely teenage girl who'd had a life-threatening infection in her younger years that left her scarred and walking with a limp. Kathy was familiar with difficult illnesses; I knew she had been brought into our lives for a reason. Now, this would be a chance for Kathy to support a friend during her illness.

Grace hadn't been to a friend's house since becoming ill three months earlier. I was concerned with how I would manage, with Grace at this friend's home about twenty minutes from our house.

I asked God for guidance in finding a balance for Grace. Grace had a difficult time every day with balancing the stimuli, medications, and homeopathic regimen. Her stamina was limited, and she was frail from being ill for three months.

I reluctantly agreed that Grace could go to Kathy's house for two hours, knowing the role of Kathy as a friend. As I drove Grace to Kathy's, I retaught her safety issues and developed a plan for her to leave if she needed to leave. Grace was to call me if she didn't feel well enough to stay. I gave Kathy my phone number as well.

I went to a local café on New Year's Eve and waited to pick up Grace. I was concerned with being farther away in case Grace suddenly did not feel well. I promptly picked up Grace at the designated time. She was ready to go home and to rest, but she'd had fun reconnecting with Kathy and her family. They had spent the two hours talking and playing on the computer.

What a special way for Grace to start a New Year, through God's grace.

JANUARY 2010

Ask and it will be given to you; seek and you will find; knock and the door will be opened to you. For everyone who asks receives; he who seeks finds, and to him who knocks, the door will be opened.—Matthew 7:7-8 NIV

With God's help and in His time, Grace continued to make progress. Progress to us was decreasing pain and increasing tolerance to activity. Four months into the journey, Grace was able to be awake more during the day. Some days she tolerated going with me on a short errand. Grace arranged her homebound school schedule around her required rest. Grace began to tolerate visits from friends for longer periods but would let her friends know when she was tired. Going outside for brief times became a goal to work toward. Grace enjoyed the snow—shoveling, sledding, and snowboarding in our yard that winter.

Our life continued to revolve around Grace's sleep, treatment regimen, appointments, and educational programs. We would try to think of a "fun" activity for each day, such as cooking a new recipe or an old favorite, which was new to Grace. Playing cards and games occasionally helped to pass the time. In reality, Grace was so exhausted that her days were full, and she would enjoy resting and chatting during most of her extra time.

The Lyme-literate specialist recommended pursuing cognitive therapy. Cognitive therapy is a psychotherapy method using problem-solving strategies to rebuild memory. Grace's total long-term memory loss was still a mystery, even to the specialist. We were sailing on uncharted waters. The objective was to treat the numerous infections in Grace's frail body. As the infections cleared, we would see what would happen with her memory.

The goal of cognitive therapy would be to make connections with the memories that Grace was recalling, possibly to other memories, which she had not recalled at this point in time. The first step would be to find a therapist trained in cognitive therapy who was willing to work with Grace's total long-term memory loss.

A family friend recommended a therapist trained in cognitive therapy. I contacted Sally, the therapist, and discussed the doctor's request. Sally was interested in meeting Grace and learning more about her illness. God had provided us with the help we needed in this next step in the journey.

In addition, we would try to get health-care insurance approval for reimbursement of cognitive therapy. After multiple phone calls with the health-care insurance company, twenty sessions of cognitive therapy were approved. I thought, *Why twenty sessions? Is there a formula used to know that twenty sessions will reach a designated, desired endpoint?*

Grace began cognitive therapy four months into the journey. Sally agreed to meet with Grace once a week. If Grace could tolerate an hour session, then that would be made available. The first few sessions lasted only slightly more than thirty minutes due to Grace's limited tolerance to being actively engaged in conversation and away from home. The first sessions were getting to know each other. Sally learned about the journey up to this point and agreed to research memory loss related to Lyme disease. She too wanted to explore the possibility of a physical or psychological assault to Grace that would have led to this amnesia.

Again, there would be no quick answers or solutions to our dilemma. Grace, however, enjoyed talking and sharing with the therapist. She was given a homework assignment to journal the slightest recall of anything during the week. Grace readily started a notepad to journal things recalled and was proud to share these things during each session.

Each session started with a recap of the events of the week with regard to Grace's illness and progress. For example, Grace would inform Sally of her headache being worse. Or Grace would talk with Sally about the homebound teacher helping her with math.

During one session, Grace relayed a memory that came back. "Uncle Bill has a beard," she told Sally.

"What else do you remember about Uncle Bill?" Sally asked.

"Nothing really," Grace sadly answered.

"Can you remember a smell?"

"No, I don't remember any smell," Grace answered quietly.

"Do you remember what his beard feels like?" Sally asked.

"No, I just know he has a beard," Grace said. Grace had not seen Uncle Bill since before she became ill.

Sally would comment to Grace and me that we were amazing to make good things out of this situation. With God's guidance, we further developed a strong mother-daughter bond. We made adventures of each day to learn and enjoy what we could for that day.

We continued to be blessed by friends and family to help us on a routine basis in managing life through this journey. God always provided just what we needed. We encouraged friends and family to send cards to Grace, which she cherished and enjoyed receiving. Grace received cards at least several times every week. As she felt better, Grace began a scrapbook with the cards sent to her. This helped her to recall her dear friends.

Our friends and family also continued to provide meals or treats periodically. One day, Grace said to me, "Remember the delicious taco dinner Virginia brought for us?"

I acknowledged the delicious meal from our friend and what a surprise it was on a difficult day. Praise be to God for our friends.

The current medical establishment does not acknowledge Lyme disease as a devastating disease or as life-threatening. Our health insurance company, fortunately, covered the first month of intravenous antibiotic treatment and then, through an appeal, agreed to cover one additional month. Without the health insurance, the cost of the medication, supplies, and infusion nurse visits would have been several thousand dollars each month.

After two months of intravenous antibiotic treatment, I was able to purchase the antibiotics in the powder form and mix them into intravenous bags for infusion. This was something I knew how to do as a nurse. Obtaining syringes to flush the intravenous line with was an obstacle—the local pharmacist did not have the size syringes that I needed. He, however, collaborated with me and was able to obtain the supplies that I would need to continue Grace's intravenous medications on a daily basis.

The winter was snowier than usual for our area. Every few days, I would spend several hours shoveling the snow off our driveway. Grace would come out to help for as long as she could, usually half an hour. Then, as any child would do, she would grab her sled and sled down our hill in the yard. One day, she asked if I could help her with her snowboard. I was nervous to let her try from the physical aspect, because of her fatigue, but also psychologically. I wanted to protect her from any pain of not being able to do something that she used to be able to do. God was with us as I helped Grace at the top of our hill by getting her feet into the snowboard. Within a minute, Grace hopped from standing forward to sideways, which is the way to start snowboarding. She was headed down the hill with a smile on her face. She was even able to stop herself. Although this was an ordinary thing for Grace at fifteen years old, I questioned how she remembered how to snowboard. Amazing Grace.

On another quiet evening at home, during dinner Grace asked if she could get the "thing that you blow through and make music." She positioned her hands as if holding her flute. She had played the flute for a few years through the school instrumental program, but how did she remember she had a flute or what a flute was? We got the flute out and immediately, Grace was able to properly position the flute and blow air through the instrument. Over the next few days, she taught herself songs from the flute again. By now, there had been a few other things that Grace was able to perform, even though her memory was gone. She had snowboarded. She had played the piano. Now, she was playing the flute. Amazing Grace, how sweet the sound.

Grace began to desire her independence and time alone when possible. I built in time in the mornings, when I would go to work, for her to be home alone. After saying many prayers, I would leave with some trepidation as Grace waved good-bye from the front door. She would quietly watch television or look at a magazine for up to an hour, before her grandmother or kid-sitter would arrive. This was a time to allow Grace to continue to develop her independence as a fifteen–year–old, within a safe range. During these times alone, Grace was safe in God's loving hands.

Even when Grace and I were home alone, she would often spend time in her bedroom, reacquainting herself with things from her past. Again, I would allow her this space and time, albeit with trepidation at times. I could hear her moving about in her bedroom, which was right above our kitchen. Sometimes, the time between hearing her move about was lengthy. I would calmly look at the clock and allow another five or ten minutes before calling up or "dropping by" her room to ask her a question. In reality, I was checking on her physical condition. Prayers were continually said and answered by God at these moments.

FEBRUARY 2010

So I tell you, whatever you ask for in prayer, believe that you have received it, and it will be yours.—Mark 11:24 NIV

Rejoice in hope, be patient in suffering, persevere in prayer.—Romans 12:12 New Oxford Annotated Bible; Oxford University Press 1994

One day, about four months into our journey, Grace mentioned, "Mom, I can't hear good out of this ear." She pointed to her right ear.

I wanted to deny the possibility that now Grace was losing her hearing. Four months into this journey, we had enough to juggle and certainly, her condition should be improving. "What do you mean you can't hear good?"

Grace explained, "I've noticed I can't hear on the phone if I hold it up to this ear."

I quickly processed this new, unexpected information.

Grace further explained, "I have been trying to hold the phone to my other ear. And that works better because I can hear then."

Not only had Grace noticed a change in her hearing, but she had investigated what she could hear from the other ear. This was definitely a clever finding on her part.

The thoughts and questions raced through my mind: *How could her hearing be gone in that ear? Is it another deficit due to Lyme disease? What will be next? Will she lose her ability to talk or to walk?*

I immediately made an appointment with her pediatrician to evaluate her hearing the following day. The hearing test showed a nearly total loss of hearing in Grace's right ear, while the left ear was functioning perfectly.

I asked the pediatrician, "Is this hearing loss related to Lyme disease?"

The pediatrician answered, "That is unclear."

"Could this be a side effect of one of Grace's medications?"

Again, the pediatrician did not give me an answer.

We were referred to an ear, nose, and throat (ENT) specialist to be further evaluated. There were so many questions with no true answers in sight. Praying was the only way to survive and to manage each day's events.

The ENT specialist confirmed that Grace had suffered nearly total hearing loss in her right ear. The ENT specialist then called Dr. L, the Lyme-literate provider, to discuss the assessment and treatment. Grace was placed on steroids for ten days.

Not only did the steroids improve her hearing, but her snapshots of memory were coming more regularly. She began to remember a long-term memory, two or three times a day, while on the steroids. Those ten days while Grace was on the steroids gave us such an inspiration of hope for her recovery from these illnesses.

After ten days, Grace and I returned to the ENT for a follow-up appointment. Grace had noticed an improvement in her hearing in her right ear. She was now able to hold the phone to her right ear and talk.

At this appointment, the hearing evaluation showed the hearing in Grace's right ear was close to 100 percent improved. I explained to the ENT the improvement in Grace's memory during these ten days, but he would not prescribe further steroids, in spite of the improvement in Grace's memory.

We had an appointment with Dr. L in the next week. I nearly begged Dr. L to allow Grace to continue on the steroids as her memory had improved notably each day. Unfortunately, staying on steroids, even a low-dose, was not recommended and not prescribed. However, Dr. L agreed to start Grace on an anti-inflammatory medication, used as an anti-malaria drug. Praise be to God—Grace's memory recall continued to progress.

I compared Grace's memory recall to a giant jigsaw puzzle. We were turning over the pieces. Each memory that returned was a piece of the jigsaw puzzle. There might be millions of pieces to turn over.

At this point, we might have turned over a hundred. This would be our journey—to continue to take whatever memories God gave Grace and keep building on those. Grace's therapist continued to recommend logging each memory as it returned. Each memory that returned was a miracle from God, a gift for us to treasure.

Grace was on her fourth month of intravenous antibiotics. Near the end of the fourth month, Grace's skin around the IV developed a rash. The skin under the intravenous dressing was breaking down. As a nurse, I knew that if the site became infected, this would be another major complication that Grace might not be able to endure.

During the next visit by the visiting IV nurse, she shifted the intravenous dressing away from most of the rash and assured us it would be okay.

A few days later, the rash continued to spread under and around the intravenous dressing. On Saturday, I took Grace to the hospital to have her IV checked.

The staff at the emergency room assessed Grace's IV and her skin. They did not feel it was necessary to discontinue the intravenous line, since it was working well. I disagreed with their assessment but was not willing to argue. My resistance was wearing down at this point.

As I administered Grace's intravenous antibiotics that evening, I was disappointed by my reluctance to insist on having Grace's IV discontinued in the ER earlier that day. Now, I noted the rash was on the insertion site of the intravenous line. I had to plan my next step, which would be to go back to the ER the next day.

Upon arriving at the emergency room, I explained the situation regarding the IV to the nurse, including our visit yesterday. As Grace's advocate, I insisted the line be discontinued to avert a likely complication.

The IV nurse for the hospital came in and discontinued the IV without any problems.

The ER informed Dr. L of the discontinued intravenous line. The following day, I called Dr. L's office to schedule an appointment to follow up. I presumed another intravenous line would be inserted in the other arm in order to continue the antibiotics.

Grace's memory was slowly returning. At this point, Grace usually remembered one or two things from the past each day.

We were able to get an appointment with Dr. L for the same day. My mother, Grace, and I made the trip to Dr. L's office.

Dr. L examined Grace's arm. She felt the skin breakdown was "a sign that we are done with the infusions for now. This is a sign that Grace's body is finished with this part of the treatment regimen."

"What? How could this be?" I asked. Thoughts raced through my mind: *She isn't cured. Her memory hasn't returned. Where is this journey going now?* "Wouldn't it be better to insert another intravenous line for further antibiotics?" I asked Dr. L.

Dr. L reassured me that the next phase would include antibiotics by mouth. The Lyme-literate specialist remained professional and calm in spite of my questioning the next steps in the treatment plan. I believed Dr. L and I were depending on God's will to be done in this journey.

MARCH 2010

When Jesus spoke again to the people, he said "I am the light of the world. Whoever follows me will never walk in darkness but will have the light of life."—John 8:12 NIV

That spring, a mission trip to Ireland we were planning to attend was approaching. Our son's school had spring-break mission trips internationally. Grace and I were planning to attend the trip, and Michael had chosen Ireland. It was a twelve-day trip involving community service in Northern Ireland. The coordinators knew about Grace's illness and accepted our making the trip, if possible. With apprehension, I continued to follow our plans for the trip. We made a poster of Ireland and learned about Ireland before the trip.

I had traveled with Grace on airplanes during her illness to visit Michael while he was attending boarding school. I had learned the issues involved with security and the ability to carry on extra fluids involved in her treatments.

Grace and I traveled to Ireland alone, not with the group, as we were leaving on different days and from different airports. We made the best of every situation and continued to learn and explore together every day. At this point, a few memories came back each day, and Grace would get to spend twelve days with her brother. Along with traveling in Ireland and being involved in community service, Grace made a lot of knew friends on the trip. There were a few events in which Grace was not feeling well enough to participate, and she would rest for the day at the hotel. International travel was tiring even for the healthy.

Apprehension mounted for me at times when Grace physically did not feel well. One day in particular, she cried and said, "I just want to go home." I would need to arrange getting back to Dublin and getting a trip home to the United States. This would not be easy. I encouraged Grace to relax for the day, and we would reevaluate in the morning. Thanks be to God, by morning she was feeling better and able to continue with the group.

One day, a few of her new friends wanted to swim in the Irish Sea. This was similar to a Polar Bear Plunge—the water temperature was chilly in mid–March in Northern Ireland. Grace hadn't been swimming since before she got sick.

I wondered, *Will she still know how?*

For years, Grace had been a competitive swimmer for her school's swim team and a summer swim team. "Will swimming come back naturally for Grace?" I asked God.

We walked down to the Irish Sea from where we were staying. Grace said, "I just want to watch them, Mom."

I knew in my heart that Grace didn't want to "just watch them."

Grace really wanted to participate. My trepidation was apparent. God would watch out for her, I knew.

I agreed and allowed Grace to plunge into the surf with her clothes on. She bobbed up and down and squealed with joy with the other teenagers. This was one of Grace's fondest memories of the trip. She swam in the Irish Sea. How many American teenagers can say that?

Eight days into the trip, my husband joined the group. We had arranged for him to come to Ireland for two days of the mission trip. He would fly home with Grace and me as the group had a few more days in Ireland. I was relieved to see him and have him as a support for the end of our trip and getting home.

"Why would you even consider taking such an ill child on a trip to this extent?" others would ask me. God had given me the support and love to continue and to be involved in the mission trip. We were able to touch others' lives, and they touched Grace's life as well. It was wonderful to watch as Grace made new friends and had new experiences. Life continued in spite of crises and illnesses. I truly believed keeping Grace involved helped her recovery. Through prayers and God's loving guidance, the trip to Ireland was a great learning experience and a wonderful mission trip to help adolescents in Northern Ireland.

APRIL 2010

So with you: Now is your time of grief, but I will see you again and you will rejoice, and no one will take away your joy.—John 16:22 NIV

Six months into our journey, we were seeing steady improvements in Grace's condition. Grace continued with the medication regimen, homeopathic treatments, cognitive therapy, and rest. Her headaches were less severe, and there were periods when she had no headache. She might have only an hour or two a day without a headache, but that was a blessing and a relief from a continuous headache. With less pain, Grace was able to concentrate for longer periods on activities.

In addition, Grace was more stable now than at any other time during this journey. Physically, she was able to do more, although not as much as a healthy, active teenage girl. Taking a short walk or swinging on a swing for fifteen minutes was a blessing to treasure. We would delight in the joy of any happiness or progress.

Grace continued to recall one to three things on most days from her long-term memory. We were encouraged to experience this progress. In this, we rejoiced, but we knew we had thousands, if not millions, more puzzle pieces to turn over and to connect. It was a daunting task, but with patience, prayers, and perseverance, we would continue on the journey that God had given to us.

As spring approached, I would take the opportunity on warmer days to walk around the neighborhood. This gave Grace chances to stay at home alone for up to half an hour. We both began to treasure these moments. Grace never enjoyed being hovered over, and during her illness she wanted some personal space.

As we spent time outside in the pleasant spring weather after a very snowy winter, we wondered if Grace would remember how to ride her bike. Frank and I decided to help Grace ride her bike one afternoon. Grace was able to ride, but she was extremely unsteady as she pedaled. This unsteadiness was likely from muscle fatigue and deconditioning. Riding her bike, however, brought smiles to Grace's face as she succeeded in doing an "old thing." Again, I wondered how she remembered to ride a bike. Amazing Grace, from God.

Along with the physical improvements, Grace was happy most of the time. She had been pleasant overall throughout this journey. Now, she was beginning to laugh and enjoy life a little at a time. God was giving us joyous moments to sustain us through the journey. Joy meant there was hope, and everybody needs hope when dealing with a catastrophic illness.

MAY 1 AND 2, 2010

I have come into the world as a light, so that no one who believes in me should stay in darkness.—John 12:46 NIV

On May 1, Grace and I went to look at open houses in the area—this had become a pastime for us on Sundays. It was a fun way to be out of the house and change the routine for a few hours. We were in the market to purchase a new home in the area, to accommodate my parents living with us as they aged. Grace and I fell in love with a house. My husband and mother were equally excited about the house, so we began the process of purchasing the house during the open house on that day. Grace was happy to find a new house for our family.

Through cognitive therapy, intravenous therapy, and homeopathic measures, we were fortunate to see Grace's progressive return of long-term memory. May 2 was a beautiful, sunny spring day. We were seven months into our journey. Grace recalled ten random memories on that day. This was the most memories that had returned in one day since this journey began. I praised God and thanked Him for each memory Grace told me.

One memory Grace recalled that afternoon was when we were outside trimming bushes in front of our house. Grace said, "I know why this bush has broken branches like this."

"What is it from, Grace?" I patiently asked.

"It is where Dad fell into the bush off of the ladder," Grace said with a smile. This was an accurate memory. Frank had fallen off the ladder into those bushes while he was hanging Christmas lights several years earlier.

This was a remarkable day for Grace's recall. I encouraged her to journal her memories. Her therapist wanted to review her journals on a weekly basis to see if connections between these memories could help Grace to recall further memories.

MAY 3, 2010

Jesus turned and saw her. "Take heart, daughter" he said,
"your faith has healed you."—Matthew 9:22 NIV

On May 3, 2010, I was preparing to leave for work on the college campus. I woke Grace, as she'd requested to go to the office with me. I would be reviewing my students' poster presentations, and Grace was interested in meeting my students as they completed their semester's work.

After waking, Grace began her morning routine of getting ready. Suddenly, she came downstairs into the kitchen and said, "Remember what the doctor said? I remember everything, Mom. Quiz me."

Wait a minute … what? Did Grace just tell me that her memory had completely returned?

Indeed, Mary, the physician's assistant, the first Lyme-literate specialist, had told us that "one day Grace's memory will all come back, just as it went away one day." We had been told this information for a reason. Yet after seven months of slow, heartbreaking progress, we were not focused on waiting for that moment to occur.

Now, here was Grace, standing in the kitchen, telling me that all of her memory was back. This was unbelievable. This was a miracle of miracles. Still, I wondered how Grace knew all of her memory was back. I had not asked her any specific questions this morning to check her memory. Was it suddenly as if she had come out of a fog and could see clearly?

With apprehension and prayers, I began asking Grace questions.

"Where does Uncle Bill live?"

"In the Florida Keys," Grace answered quickly and with certainty.

"What is your favorite ride at Disney World?"

"Space Mountain!" Grace answered.

Grace was able to answer accurately each question that I asked. With tears in my eyes, I continued to explore the memories that had returned. I was concerned about asking questions that Grace might not be able to answer. However, as each moment went by, I realized the dream had come true. Our prayers had been answered. Grace's total long-term memory had returned overnight.

We had lived through each day making the best of each moment that God gave us. If Mary had told us, "In seven months, her memory will come back," would we have experienced the same journey? We had been on the journey, and God had carried us and protected us each moment along the way. Thanks be to God for this miracle.

We continued with our morning preparation to go to the college. During our half-hour drive to the campus, I had Grace make phone calls to her father, her brother, her grandparents, and her uncle and aunt.

Each call started with Grace's saying, "Hi, this is Grace. Guess what happened?"

"I don't know. What happened?" came the response on the other end of the phone.

Grace gleefully cried out, each time, "My memory came back this morning!"

With tears and cheers and prayers of thanksgiving, Grace was able to tell her family that she now remembered each of them. She knew who they were and what their personalities were like. She now remembered the things her friends and family liked to do, what made them laugh, and what they liked to do with her. All of this had been lost on that October morning, seven months ago.

I placed a call to Angela during our drive to campus and told her I had exciting news. "Grace's memory came back this morning!" I cried out to her. She had been our angel throughout this journey. She was a prayer warrior for Grace.

"What?" Angela cried.

"Yes, Angela, everything came back when she woke up this morning," I explained.

"Linda, that makes sense."

"Angela, how does this make any sense at all?"

"I spent my day yesterday in prayerful fasting. I have tried to do this before, but I have never made it through a whole day in prayerful fasting. I knew during the day that I was praying for somebody but I didn't know who it was." As a strong Christian woman, Angela was driven to further develop her faithful life. I knew about her experiences with prayerful fasting. This was a practice that she had decided to pursue.

"When I broke my fast this morning, I knew that something had happened. Then, you called me."

Angela and I rejoiced in prayer for the miracle that God had delivered.

Praise of thanksgiving poured over our existence.
Believe me when I say that I am in the Father and the Father is in me; or at least believe on the evidence of miracles themselves.—John 14:11 NIV

COPING

Come to me, all you that are weary and are carrying heavy burdens, and
I will give you rest. Take my yoke upon you, and learn from me; for I
am gentle and humble in heart, and you will find rest for your souls. For
my yoke is easy, and my burden is light.—Matthew 11:28-30 NIV

From the very first day, I believed God gave this journey to us because He believed in us. We were strong enough to make the journey together, with God's help through our family and friends. Our faith was strong and would only get stronger with such a journey.

I quickly realized that above everything else, I was an advocate for Grace. As a registered nurse, I developed knowledge to get us through this journey, which will help others. Through this journey, I also became an advocate to others with Lyme disease and other tick-borne diseases.

Through this journey, I never questioned God with "why me?" I prayed for strength and courage each day. I prayed for guidance and love. I did question "why Grace?" Sometimes, our questions were not clearly answered by God right away. Fortunately, God gave Grace an inner strength superior to most people and a high pain tolerance. In addition, Grace was not a complainer. These were characteristics that made a difficult journey more tolerable for each of us.

Another coping mechanism often stated by parents, especially mothers, is "I'd rather be in your shoes than to see you suffer." I never had this thought. In reality, I did often think about if the circumstances had been changed. What if I'd had a sudden long-term memory loss like Grace? The medical profession may have easily diagnosed me with early-onset dementia, early Alzheimer's disease. They would have prescribed medications for this and told my family to enjoy the years that we could.

During our journey with Lyme disease, Grace attended my Bible study group each week. Even on days when she wasn't feeling her best, she would quietly ask me to take her to the Bible study. Prayers were offered up for her and her healing. In addition, Grace was on prayer lists in many communities, as news of her illness and suffering spread. Knowing others cared and were praying was an immense relief to me every day. Grace attended weekly church services as well. Again, even though getting up in the morning when she didn't feel well was difficult, Grace would quietly insist that we get to church. Prayers were offered up for her and her healing each week at church as well.

Through intercessory prayers—the practice of praying for others—miracles happened. Sometimes, that is all that you can do. Sometimes you can't change the issue others are facing, but you can pray. Sometimes you can't do anything specifically to help others, especially when you are not in close proximity to the ill person, but you can pray. People may ask if praying is all that they can do. Real prayers do help. Prayers are answered by God.

Grace got into the routine of saying to me, "Don't worry; don't be sad. It is all going to okay." This was especially hard as I tried to deal with the enormity of this journey and the everyday management of the treatment regimen. From the voice of a child, we need to learn life's lessons. She was the sick one, ministering to me.

Learning and remembering to smile whenever possible became paramount to our everyday lives together. Most people may only see the suffering and pain and not the joy of this journey. A smile means a lot to people who see it. A smile also means a lot to the person smiling.

I would smile as Grace relearned facts and tasks. Then I would smile a bigger smile when a memory came back. Her memories tended to return out of the blue. In the middle of an activity, Grace would remember a random memory. Those were moments that always brought a smile for me. Each smile meant a ray of new hope in this journey.

Each morning, I would smile as Grace woke up. Hearing her talk and remember the things she learned the day before made me smile. I found myself laughing more than usual as we learned things together.

I also found time to reflect on other people we would see during our appointments or errands. This world has a lot of people experiencing a lot of stress. As somebody cut me off as we drove to have an MRI performed on Grace, I smiled and said he must have a lot on his mind. I chose to cherish every moment that God gave to us.

As our journey continued I would take time for my health. I am an avid walker and was actually preparing for a three-day sixty-mile Breast Cancer Walk when Grace got sick. As time permitted, I would take a walk for a few miles in our neighborhood. Remember to take care of the caretaker. Yes, that may be you.

Being outside was healthy for me. I loved working outside in the yard or shoveling snow. At the beginning of our journey, it was autumn. I would take half an hour or an hour each day to rake leaves. Grace learned how to rake leaves and to jump in the piles of leaves again. Smelling the fragrance of leaves and fall was refreshing. Often, however, Grace would stay inside to rest while I went outside.

Another way I took care of the caretaker was to rest whenever I could. I did not have nearly as many errands to run and places to go, so there was more time at home than usual. Relaxing with a book or handwork or a movie was a welcome break. I also practiced mindful meditation, which helped me to refocus my attention on God. Sleeping at night was frequently disrupted due to Grace's discomfort, but we would sleep when we could. The chaotic days of school and sports were gone. There was a relaxing aspect to this major change in our lifestyle. Rather than tormenting myself over why something had to be a certain way, I enjoyed the differences and the time at home.

Eating healthy was something else I did for myself during the journey. The stress of Grace's illness and the uncertainty in my life led to a decreased appetite for me. I focused on eating healthy food. In reality, I lost several pounds throughout the difficult months.

One last thing I found helpful was to verbalize my experiences with those close to me. My Bible study friends, family members, and neighbors were great at listening when I wanted to talk, and they respected my desire to be quiet when I needed it. We gave praise to the Lord and abundant thanks for God's loving support. Daily, we thanked God for family and friends; without them, the journey of Grace's memory loss and severe headaches would have been impossible.

BEFORE OCTOBER FIRST

Jesus said: "But this happened so that the work of God might be displayed in his life."—John 9:3 NIV

Maybe there were signs of Grace's illness before the first day of this journey. Hindsight was always 20/20. As we reviewed everything that had been going on with Grace for the last few weeks, months, and possibly even for years, possible connections were revealed.

First, we knew that two months prior to her total long-term memory loss, she was diagnosed with Lyme disease. It was August, and she had a cold. She didn't feel well at all—a lot of congestion, fever, and body aches. Within a few days, she had multiple discolorations over her entire body. These were in circle formations and several inches in diameter. These spots had redness in the center and were paler toward their edges. Each day, as the heat of the summer day increased, Grace's spots would become more defined, deeper in color, and more uncomfortable. During the night, they would nearly disappear. I had never seen any skin rash like this before, as a nurse or as a mother. After several days of these spots, I decided to take her to the pediatrician. Grace was diagnosed with Lyme disease and prescribed three weeks of doxycycline, an antibiotic. Her symptoms improved slowly, and by the end of August, she did feel better, and the spots, which were the bull's-eyes, did go away.

Grace was properly diagnosed at that time with Lyme disease but no other infections. She was treated with the proper medication but just not for long enough, according to the Lyme-literate physician. Grace was not misdiagnosed; she was undertreated at that point. In addition, no other infections were diagnosed in August.

Another hindsight was that we also had Grace in the emergency room earlier in the summer because she woke up one night and called for me. She said she was having problems breathing. I comforted her and sat with her for a few minutes. I actually went back to bed for a few minutes but then realized that was very strange. Why would she suddenly be short of breath? I got back out of bed and took her to the ER. They noted a skin rash at that time, but they did not make a diagnosis related to her shortness of breath. In hindsight, this was very likely related to the Lyme disease infection.

Another strange thing had happened six months prior to our "first day." Grace and I had taken a power walk through our neighborhood. I was training for a three-day Breast Cancer Walk. Grace had decided to join me and get some exercise. During the latter part of the walk, Grace complained of her knee hurting. It began to hurt so bad that she was unable to walk the rest of the distance back to our house. I left her in a neighbor's yard and went to get the car. I drove her home as the pain was too great. I took her to the ER the next day, and they were unable to determine any physical damage to her knee. Likely, this could have been related to Lyme disease as well.

As we put the different scenarios together afterward, this led us to believe Grace was likely infected with Lyme disease (and possibly the other infections) for an extended period. How would we have known an episode of shortness of breath was Lyme disease? How would we know a knee that hurt after exercising was Lyme disease? I don't think anybody would have put the diagnosis of either of these as Lyme disease, but they are symptoms likely related to the infection.

Before the first day of our journey, Grace was often irritable and often chose not to be physically active. We thought this was her personality developing as a teenager. However, this could have been due to her being ill and not feeling well.

Questions that we asked that have not been answered were:

- o Was it possible that she was so sick with the multiple infections that her brain just decided it had enough and had to stop?
- o Was that why she lost her long-term memory, as part of the stress on her body?

o If not treated, would the infections have continued until they killed her?

Through God's loving hands, Grace was home and safe when she lost her memory, and thanks be to God for carrying us through the proper diagnosis of the multiple infections and receiving the medical treatment Grace needed to stay alive here on earth.

ASKING FOR HELP

In everything I [Paul] did, I showed you that by this kind of hard work
we must help the weak, remembering the words the Lord Jesus himself
said: "It is more blessed to give than to receive."—Acts 20:35 NIV

A lesson we each can learn is to help others when they are in a crisis. Be specific. Wonderful memories came from our friends during this difficult journey. We still talk about some of the great things our friends did during that time.

Doing something for those who are ill and those who are shut-ins does make a difference in their lives and in yours, too. A few moments of time can really make a difference. Since our journey began, I've been asked advice on what to do to help others in our community who are sick. The best answer is to do *something*. Doing nothing is not helpful. A simple note to the person or the family is a blessing. A specific day and time that you are available to sit with the ill person while the family runs errands or your running the errands is a blessing. Making a meal is a blessing. You may have to step outside of your box, but you will be glad that you did. God will be glad that you did. You are to follow Jesus's examples. In turn, others will follow your examples as well.

This was a beautiful part of the journey. These people stepped outside of their comfort zone to reach out and to help. I had a list of people I could call for different days of the week and the times they were available.

A year and a half after the beginning of the journey, several relatives commented to me that they could not personally visit from out-of-state while Grace was so ill. My dearest uncle would inquire frequently as to Grace's progress, but he could not bear the thought of seeing her while being seriously ill. Grace would not have recognized him, and he personally knew he could not face this situation. Then my aunt said on a visit that she purposely did not visit when Grace was seriously ill, as she knew she could not see Grace so sick. I know the same was true of some other acquaintances in the community. They would hear the story through my friends and family but never offer assistance or visit. I recall an acquaintance in the community seeing me nearly five months into our journey. She stated she had heard about Grace being sick and asked how she was doing. Yet she did not call or e-mail or drop a note to us to let us know she was thinking about us. I then realized that some people have not learned to give in a godly manner. I continue to pray for people to reach out and help others in some way every day. We, as Christians, need to strengthen our ability to help others. Our discomfort with the situation may be a reality, but God wants us to reach out to those in need.

AFTERWORD

*The beginning of wisdom is this: Get wisdom; and whatever
else you get, get insight.*—Proverbs 4:7 New Oxford
Annotated Bible; Oxford University Press 1994

Contemporary alternative methods are employed by people with illness to address their symptoms beyond traditional medicine. When patients utilize the alternative measures, traditional medical practitioners may not agree with their efficacy. This was certainly the case with our journey.

When we sought medical attention for everyday situations, most frequently the physicians would say something along the lines of "How much longer are you planning on doing this?" How unnerving to be questioned by a professional about the treatment you have chosen, especially for your child. We were also told by physicians that the specialists were just taking our money and that we should be cautious.

Remember, we sought the specialist after multiple traditional physicians could not diagnose any physical problem with Grace. We were indeed desperate for some answers. We were ready for a diagnosis. We were ready for a treatment plan. It made sense, when she'd been diagnosed with six infections, that she needed treatment to kill the infecting organisms. Why would a traditional physician or an insurance company ever question the efficacy of this treatment?

Maybe nobody could say for certain why Grace lost all of her long-term memory one night. Maybe it never had been documented before. But it did happen. And Grace did have six infections in her body at one time. The traditional medical professionals couldn't find the infections. Not with the laboratories they used. Not in her blood. Not in her cerebrospinal fluid. Not evidenced on a CAT scan. Not evidenced on an EEG. Not evidenced on an MRI.

Be aware the conditions can exist. Vigilance was the key to getting a diagnosis and then getting treatment. I wondered how many people had been diagnosed with a psychiatric illness that might have been a treatable infection.

I have never been so guided and carried by our Lord as I was during this journey. Turning everything over to God was a powerful experience.

We truly experienced amazing moments in a crazy time. We witnessed miracles. We experienced a multitude of blessings—God provided us with happy times with happy memories.

You will be called upon to be an advocate for your family member or for yourself throughout your life. For me, being an advocate for Grace involved seeking advice from multiple resources: physicians, physician's assistants, nurses, psychiatrists, psychologists, friends, family members, others with similar circumstances, and literature. Gathering information was crucial, overwhelming, and scary. Hearing the nightmares of others often led to feelings of hopelessness and fear.

Prayer for guidance and support was crucial. You will be called to follow your heart in making decisions, even if the decisions may not be the most popular route. God will give you the answers throughout your journey, but you have to listen. God continually guided us each day and even each hour. Don't settle for something you know isn't right. This was hard when the authorities were telling me something I didn't believe. This happened numerous times during our journey. Recall that we did not settle for Grace being admitted to the psychiatric ward at the Children's Hospital. The neurology team advised inpatient psychiatric treatment for this sudden loss of long-term memory. In addition, we were told that Grace had "too many positive gains" from being at home, a few weeks into our journey. We were advised to send her back to middle school, so she could face her problems. In reality, at that time we did not know Grace had six infections in her body. However, I knew that sending her back to her school was not facing her problems. Be cautious of advice that doesn't seem to work for your situation.

The school district continued to support Grace's education on homebound instruction for eight months. The nurse and the counselor from her school offered several times for Grace to visit the school.

We took a tour of the school within two months of the onset of this illness, but Grace was not able to recall anything about the school: rooms, lockers, teachers, or the cafeteria. She certainly was not ready to return to school at this point. The counselor offered for her to meet a few of her friends at the school for lunch in the guidance office. However, Grace was never quite up to making the lunch date. With God by our side, Grace was able to complete ninth grade. She had attended only five weeks of school before becoming gravely ill. We are fortunate and thankful for the support of the school district during such a difficult time.

God led us to and provided us with health-care providers to diagnose Grace's condition. Learning as much as we could about these diagnoses and organisms became imperative to our journey.

Even when the physicians' advice was contrary to my inner knowledge and soul, I continued to follow God's words. I continued to ask for guidance every step in this journey.

We had a few isolated days when Grace's headache returned in the first year since her memory returned. These were scary, unsettling, and nerve-racking times. The first "bad day," Grace woke up with a severe headache and was unable to communicate clearly. She was not confused. She just couldn't get her thoughts into words. She was totally frustrated and scared. This day followed a weekend when she had been very busy with very little sleep. Her headache was in the same location as it had been when this journey started. We quickly transported her to the Lyme-literate specialist, an hour and a half away from our home. The specialist alerted us that this would likely happen when Grace was fatigued. But what should we do about the severe headache? Motrin was not helping.

The Lyme-literate specialist offered peppermint oil, rubbed on the base of Grace's neck and on her temples. Then, Grace softly inhaled the scent. Within two minutes, Grace's headache disappeared, and she was able to communicate clearly again. This was another miracle. This was a true blessing. God had blessed the Lyme-literate specialist with the knowledge of the healing powers of peppermint oil.

The aromatherapy of peppermint oil dilates the blood vessels. Increasing the blood flow to the brain releases the tension involved in this type of headache. As a homeopathic, non-pharmaceutical approach, Grace was able to carry the peppermint oil with her to school without repercussions. This allowed her to manage her disease on an individual basis and as a maturing young lady. Although the headaches are frightful when they occur, God has given us the patience to realize these are just minor setbacks in the big scheme of Grace's life and her recovery.

Do not worry about tomorrow, for tomorrow will bring worries of
its own. Today's trouble is enough for today.—Matthew 6:34
New Oxford Annotated Bible; Oxford University Press 1994

A year after the beginning of the journey, Grace had her memory back for five months. Her Lyme disease was classified as chronic, and she will need to keep her immune system strong for the rest of her life. Flare-ups in Lyme disease might happen.

A year after Grace's memory came back was a milestone. During this year, Grace had three incidents when she was exhausted, with difficulty expressing herself. *Expressive aphasia* is the medical term. Each of these incidents involved a headache and exhaustion. Once she slept and got the headache to go away, she was able to clearly express herself. Three tough days in one year isn't bad for a chronic illness, I guess. This has become a new philosophy for my daily life.

Grace is a very active and involved teenage girl. She has a part-time job and is active on a crew team. She is learning to drive. She is dreaming of going away to college in two more years. She has been on several trips through school and managed herself very well. She has homeopathic and prescription medications that keep her strong and healthy. She wants to be independent.

I often wonder if Lyme disease will ever make her that sick again. The journey continues. I rest assured that God has kept her safe. With any incident she has experienced, she has gotten help immediately. The Lyme-literate specialist says these incidents are nowhere near where we were at the beginning of the journey.

Grace is a happier person now than ever before. Before being diagnosed, she was often anxious about everyday life and events. The illness has released her from that anxiety and worry. She doesn't worry about very much these days. She actually has written a "bucket list" with dreams she'd like to come true during her life. This sixteen-year-old has a real focus on things she wants to accomplish and do before the end of her life. I don't think there are too many teenagers with this perspective on their lives. She says she doesn't want to live her life in fear. She doesn't want to do anything stupid and careless, but she wants to enjoy any adventure she can during her life.

Facing death and illness at a young age was a challenge. Yet Grace has grown through being ill and enjoys life tremendously.

I often think of all the children with chronic illness and life-threatening illnesses. Diabetes, asthma, epilepsy, and autism are a few chronic illnesses that parents and children have to manage every day. Cancer, organ transplants, and severe allergic reactions are life-threatening conditions that other parents and children manage every day. Parents develop coping mechanisms to live life to the fullest with their children. God provides the strength to live life this way.

Living with Lyme disease as a chronic illness changes your perspective on life. Life is precious and sweet. Life is unpredictable and can be taken away from us at a moment's notice.

Today, I realize that a family member could leave our home today and not return, due to a fatal car accident. Living life now brings an appreciation for every day that God gives us to live it to the fullest.

Others have done the hard work, and you have reaped
the benefits of their labor.—John 4:38 NIV

Frustration exists since the medical community and the health insurance companies will not recognize the symptoms of Lyme disease. They do not believe symptoms so severe are related to Lyme disease. Only through a Lyme-literate specialist can full treatment be provided, but the health insurance companies will not compensate for this treatment, because they are not part of the standard medical protocols. What do the physicians and health-care insurance companies fear? Do they fear losing control? Is it about money? How can they continually turn their heads away from an illness that has reached epidemic levels in the United States? Why is the medical profession refusing to recognize this disease?

I think about the turn of events and how many people are likely infected with Lyme disease and not aggressively treated. Are there people in the psychiatric units who are infected? Are there people diagnosed with Alzheimer's who are infected? The literature identified the possibility that many cases of multiple sclerosis may be related to Lyme disease. Take a moment to think about the implications for so many infected people. Lyme disease and babeiosis are tick-borne diseases that are not diagnosed early and not adequately treated.

A vaccination for Lyme disease was on the market but was discontinued. Our animals can receive a Lyme disease vaccine, but humans can't.

Tick-borne diseases can be debilitating and life-threatening. Thirty years ago, our country faced a new, unknown virus. The medical community did not know what was causing people to be so ill and die so quickly. This disease became known as human immunodeficiency virus (HIV), which becomes AIDS as the virus infects the human body with various infections while it is weakened by HIV. The medical community quickly researched the virus causing this new illness. Diagnostic tests were identified and treatment protocols were researched and funded. In the beginning of this epidemic HIV/AIDS was indeed a death sentence to anybody infected. Over the next decades, medicines were developed and protocols established to treat people infected with HIV. Delaying the onset of infections in the weakened bodies of those infected with HIV has become hallmark to their survival.

Why the big push to find a diagnosis and treatment for HIV/AIDS? HIV is spread through blood and body secretions. One impetus for the efforts with HIV/AIDS was our society's blood supply was in jeopardy of further spreading this virus.

Babeiosis can be transmitted through blood transfusions. The FDA is currently working on screening blood for babeiosis in the blood donated in this country. Why are the tick-borne diseases not as important in establishing a medically accepted protocol for treatment? Why is the funding not available to pursue this diagnostic and treatment protocols that is so needed by anybody suffering from Lyme disease or babeiosis? These infections are treatable. We live in a society with the capability to properly diagnose and treat these infections.

Perhaps having celebrities or well-known people diagnosed with a tick-borne infection would begin the prospects of moving these tick-borne infections to the forefront.

Interestingly enough, Grace now recalls that she did not feel well for a very long time, perhaps years before our journey began. She recalls feeling sick every day of middle school—for two years. She remembers having headaches nearly every day for those years. Why didn't we know she felt so badly? She thought it was the way her life was going to be. She says she never felt well. Nobody even knew how terrible she felt. How sad for a teenager to feel sick.

> *My Father will give you whatever you ask in my name. Until now you have not asked for anything in my name. Ask and you will receive, and your joy will be complete.—John 16:23-24 NIV*

MAKING A DIFFERENCE

*Ask and you will receive, so that your joy may
be complete.—John 16:24 NIV*

Three years have passed since Grace's memory returned. We have
been so blessed through God with His miracles and with guidance
throughout this journey. The journey did not end when Grace's memory
returned. The journey will continue, now in a way to help others. God
commands us to help others and to love our neighbors.

I learned an extraordinary amount of information along this journey.
Before Grace became gravely ill, I had heard of Lyme disease and knew
it was from infected deer ticks, but I did not know the difficulty of
getting diagnosed or the severity of the illness.

I had personally heard from park rangers at a local county park,
"Don't worry about Lyme disease because it only comes from deer
ticks." In addition, the park rangers would say, "The ticks that you may
see on you do not have Lyme disease." Looking back, those statements
scare me. Not even those people trained in the parks services provided
appropriate information.

Our children have always been active and chose to be outside
as long as possible when the weather permitted. Grace was infected
from deer ticks. Staying inside possibly would have prevented those
infections, but she preferred to be outdoors.

I truly cannot believe that I did not know enough to take preventive
steps to avoid Lyme disease in our family and in our community.
I believed if somebody got infected, there would be a diagnosis,
treatment, and cure.

God gave us this journey for a reason. I am being called to promote
Lyme disease prevention. Just as sunburn, for example, is preventable,

Lyme disease is preventable. People do not have to stay inside to avoid Lyme disease; precautions can be taken—avoid wooded areas, wear long sleeves and long pants, apply spray to repel deer ticks, and check for ticks on your body every day. In addition, when coming in from outside, take a shower within three hours. Recall, the deer tick that transmits Lyme disease is no bigger than the period at the end of this sentence. Vigilance in prevention is essential to avoid becoming infected.

Educating those in the community in preventive measures can save a life and prevent suffering. Promoting products that repel deer ticks would further promote prevention of Lyme disease.

As the crisis mode of this journey has lessened, daily life now is more normal. It has been three years since Grace's memory returned, and she is a very happy and healthy teenager, ready for college next year as a freshman. She has the normal need to be independent. Grace takes supplements to maintain a healthy immune system and to prevent migraine headaches. On the three-year anniversary of the beginning of this journey, Grace wrote a note to us. Here is an excerpt:

> Thinking back three years ago, I woke up remembering nothing. I was a sick little kiddo. As I get older and get over my sickness, I've realized that I would still be just as sick (probably sicker) if it wasn't for you guys. Thank you so much for supporting me and making sure I got the proper care. I know several people that have been in Foundations and other psych places. I'm glad I wasn't sent to one of them. Not a day goes by without me thinking about my whole experience.

My role in the journey will not ever be completed. Through God, I have been given this experience as a mom and as a registered nurse to be an advocate for others infected with Lyme disease. I offer encouragement and insight to those infected and suffering through the disease process. I pray I will be able to inform others of the dangers of tick-borne diseases from prevention and through treatment. Prevention and early detection may be the key to slowing the impact of this disease in our country. Proper diagnosis and treatment can save the lives of the victims. God is providing us with the ability to help others through our prayers and knowledge. May we trust in God and be His servants.

Praise be to God for all of our blessings.

ANGELA AS OUR PRAYER WARRIOR

Looking back to when we first found out Grace had lost most of her memory makes me stop and ponder how far we have come since then and what brought us to this place today, where we feel the need to write about it. It was indeed an honor to be asked if I would contribute to this book that I believe will have a life-changing effect on the many people into whose hands this book will fall. For some it will be health that will be restored and for others, it is my sincere prayer that their hearts will be touched and changed by reading about this miracle; there just is no other explanation for what transpired.

Sitting in the emergency room that morning, knowing I had been summoned to provide support to Grace and Linda, I felt the need to pray as I was waiting to hear if there was any news as to why Grace had lost her memory. The memory of that day had been swirling around in my head, and I was trying to understand how Grace could have been fine the day before but awakened the next day in total confusion.

We were all at Bible study when we found out what had happened and were asked to pray for Grace. It was hard for any of us to believe what was described to us: Grace did not even know how to turn on the faucet in the bathroom. It was a relief to know that her mother was a nurse, and she would know how to proceed. It was also important for us to all do what we knew could bring about the best change, and that was to pray. Our Bible study group's name is the Mustard Seeds, and we had seen mountains moved in the past through prayer. So as I sat in the emergency room, praying once again, it was that memory that took me right back to the place where we left off praying at Bible study. I remember tuning everything out and just praying that we would find out what was wrong with Grace and that she would be healed.

I had not been praying very long when I could hear the small, still voice I often hear in prayer whisper, "Tell them to check for Lyme disease." I stopped praying and asked the nurse at the desk if I could go back for a few minutes to speak with Linda. She allowed me to go, and I could see Linda standing in the doorway of Grace's small emergency room cubicle. I told her what I heard while I was praying, and I asked that she would make sure they tested her for Lyme disease before we left the hospital. At that time, there were many tests being run, but none were conclusive. Linda assured me she would have her tested. I was relieved and headed back to the waiting room.

I had experienced Lyme disease just three years before this, and I was misdiagnosed; the additional pain I experienced because of the additional time I had this disease due to the misdiagnosis was often unbearable. I had to go on antibiotics for four months, far longer than if we had known what it was earlier. Even after that, it took many months before I felt totally healed. All of those symptoms started to flood my thoughts: headaches, the thinning of my hair, blurred vision, ringing in my ears, sore throats, confusion and difficulty in thinking, heart palpitations, stiffness in my joints and especially in my right hip, leg cramps, and foot pain. The pain in my feet caused me to actually change my footwear so my feet would not hurt so badly. My other shoes sat abandoned on my shelf, because wearing them was just too painful. All of these symptoms, along with feeling tired much of the time, resulted in my searching for the truth of what was going on with my body. I just knew something was terribly wrong, and I was getting worse instead of feeling better after seeing the doctor. I had mentioned a red oblong mark on my neck; that led the doctor to believe it was an outbreak of shingles.

My research finally led me to a website for Lyme disease, and it had all the symptoms that I was experiencing listed. I was so excited, because I really thought this was what I had experienced now for close to six months. I gathered all my research, created a folder for it, and called the doctor's office to schedule a new appointment. My doctor listened very carefully, and after reviewing all my symptoms and the materials I had gathered and taking into consideration that I had been feeling bad for so long, he suggested that we should start the antibiotics that treat Lyme disease right away. It saddened me to know how long I would have to stay on the medicine. If I had been treated right away, the treatment time would have been much shorter, and I would not have gotten all those debilitating symptoms. There was no time to look backward, though; what was done was done, and I just wanted to hope this was an accurate diagnosis. I was convinced now that it was Lyme disease. I just wanted to be well again.

My thoughts were interrupted by Linda's coming to tell me they were finishing the discharge papers for Grace, and she thought it would be best to take Grace to the Children's Hospital for more testing. The hospital we were in had discharged her without any diagnosis, and we both felt we needed answers and should head to the Children's Hospital. I asked if they had tested for Lyme, and they had not, because they did not think it could Lyme-related. We all needed to regroup, but I really wanted to stay with them and continue to pray. We decided quickly that we would go home and gather some items we might need. It felt like we were going to be in for a long evening, so we wanted to be prepared. Linda told me she would pick me up at my home, and we could drive down to the hospital together.

On the way to the Children's Hospital, Grace was actually in good spirits, and I was so amazed at how calm and accommodating she was with my being there, since she couldn't remember who I was. Linda was also very calm and confident that we would get a correct diagnosis. I had known Linda for a long time and knew she was a woman of great faith. The ride was very pleasant, but getting Grace help dominated our thoughts. It took nearly an hour to get there, but it seemed so much longer than that.

It was getting late, and we were thrilled to see that not many people were waiting to be seen when we got there. They took Grace quickly back to triage and then immediately into an emergency room cubicle. I just started praying again and really was asking for guidance and wisdom for the doctors, and then I heard the very same whisper: "Tell them to check for Lyme disease." I know this voice well, and I knew our prayers were being answered. I was excited to tell Linda that I heard the very same thing while I was praying and to please have her tested. We were there for quite some time, but there was no definitive diagnosis, and Linda was to follow up with her physician if there was no change. I was so saddened when they didn't listen and perform a test for Lyme. I just remember feeling somewhat numb on the way home, and I couldn't imagine how Grace or Linda must have felt. We just didn't have much to say on the way home. It was close to two in the morning when they dropped me off. I slipped into bed next to my husband, who was already sleeping, and my heart just ached. I just thought about how frightened and confused Grace must have felt, knowing both hospitals had no answers. I was exhausted and quickly fell into a deep dreamless sleep.

That next morning, I just couldn't get Grace off my mind, so I prayed for help: I felt the same small voice guiding me to call Linda and to give her the name of the Lyme specialist that had treated another friend of mine, a doctor who was an advocate of the accurate diagnosis of Lyme disease. I was also directed to make sure Grace's blood was tested at the lab this doctor used in California. I got so excited that I couldn't wait to speak to Linda. When I called, I was just hoping she would have good news, and there would be a change, but there was none. I shared with her all the information I had, and she said she was going to contact this doctor right away, and I knew she would. I felt so calm, and I thanked God so much for answering our prayers.

Several weeks later, it was confirmed that Grace had Lyme disease and several other infections. She was going to have to start IV treatments of antibiotics to combat this disease. We were so thankful that the tests came back with a positive diagnosis, because now she could start being treated. I couldn't help falling to my knees and just thanking the Lord for such clear direction and for the blessing of now knowing how to proceed.

Linda quickly moved into the action plan of what must be done medically for Grace. There were just so many hurdles that she had to jump through in order to get the medication Grace needed covered by insurance. I marveled at Linda's patience and determination to do everything she needed to do so that Grace had all she needed to recover. In the midst of all those preparations, Linda also had to make preparations for Grace to be homeschooled.

It was a long journey to recovery, and we prayed constantly. Those of us who stuck close by this family's side knew this journey would someday turn into something positive, where others would benefit from Grace's battle with Lyme disease. Linda let us all know at Bible study one day that she had started research in the area of Lyme disease, and it had been brought to her attention the large number of cases that are misdiagnosed, ultimately causing many to suffer unnecessarily. A Lyme disease advocate was being born. Her background in nursing, her faith, and her ability to stay calm and focused qualified her for this challenge.

These were difficult and challenging times for all of us who were watching Grace relearn just the basics, like tying a shoelace or opening a door. It broke our hearts when she would stand confused sometimes, because she couldn't figure something out, and she didn't want to bother anyone. She stayed as sweet as ever, but became childlike in some ways. I was so inspired by not ever seeing her angry or bitter. I did know she was struggling at times at home and became discouraged at times, but I wondered if I could have walked with as much grace as she did during that entire time. She was always a young person who seemed to have an old soul full of wisdom.

I remember visiting her one day with a bag of goodies that might cheer her up. Linda told me we would have to visit with Grace in the basement, because it was dark and quiet down there. She explained that Grace had been having severe headaches, and this environment was the best place for her during these headaches. Sometimes they would last for days. It made me feel so good to know how many people were sending her cards, visiting, bringing food by the house, and just showing how much they cared. I know this blessed Linda as well. Grace's dad was a pilot, and I didn't get to see him often during this time, but I knew all these gestures of kindness touched his heart as well.

Months had gone by, and we gathered and prayed for Grace each week. We prayed that her entire memory would return. As time went on, however, we wondered if her memory would ever return. She was learning old things and new things so quickly but was not able to recall the past—it could be so frustrating.

It was approximately six months after her diagnosis that I was reading a book on prayer and fasting. I was amazed at what happened in the Bible as I read all the accounts of combining prayer and fasting and the results that were unleashed because of it. There was Esther, the queen of Persia, who called for all the Jews to join her in a solemn fast for three days, because the life of her people was hanging in the balance (Esther 4:16). Anna was a faithful servant and prophetess who dedicated her life to prayer and fasting night and day (Luke 2:37). Cornelius, the Roman centurion, stated, "Four days ago I was fasting until this hour: and at the ninth hour I prayed in my house, and behold, a man stood before me in bright clothing and said, 'Cornelius, your prayer has been heard, and your alms are remembered in the sight of God'" (Acts 10:30-31). Amazing and miraculous things happened.

I was almost three-quarters of the way through the book when I heard the small whisper again say, "Fast on liquids only tomorrow for one day." I had never fasted before, but I knew I was supposed to do this even, though I didn't understand why. That next day, I prayed and fasted. I had learned that Jesus himself affirmed in Luke 5:35 that after His death, fasting would be appropriate for His followers. Spiritual fasting clearly has a place and a purpose for God's people today. It was a quiet day, full of prayer. Grace and many others were included in my prayers that day. Mainly, my desire that day was to be obedient to that small voice that asked me to pray and fast.

I woke up early the following morning, and the first thing on my mind was yesterday's day of prayer and fasting and wondering what that was about. But I needed to run a few errands that morning, so my thoughts quickly turned to what I needed to do. When I returned home, there was a message from Linda, saying she had really good news. I called immediately. Linda told me that Grace had gotten her full memory back. We were both giddy with excitement. Then, I suddenly remembered my learning about the power of prayer and fasting and the fact that I actually had done that very thing just the day before.

I told Linda about it; she called Grace to the phone, and I told her the story as well. I asked her how her memory had returned, and she said that yesterday (the day I had prayed and fasted) chunks of information returned throughout the day, and by this morning, all her memory was restored. I thought about how I had been fasting and praying that whole day, the day her memory was returning in bits and pieces. Her full memory had been restored by the following morning, which was when I broke my fast. We celebrated all over again and just thanked God for this miracle. In addition to the miracle of Grace's memory returning, the Lord apparently had just shown us the incredible power of prayer and fasting. That day will never leave me. It is one of those moments that is etched in my memory forever. It increased my faith, and I was overcome with joy and gratitude.

When Linda asked me to write this chapter of the book, I was indeed grateful for the opportunity. One thing dominated my thoughts when I sat down to write, and that was that God would get the glory for healing Grace. I prayed, and He answered with the proper diagnosis. Linda was obedient in believing this answer and going to the doctor and using the laboratory we were directed to use—all through hearing and being obedient to that small voice that spoke during prayer. Grace was treated with antibiotics and ultimately healed during the day I was called to fast and pray.

That small voice I have referenced is the voice of the Holy Spirit that lives in the heart of believers in Jesus Christ. It is my prayer that no matter who you are and what you have believed before you read this book that you will get to know who Jesus is and accept His invitation of grace through faith.

So what is faith?

F Is for Forgiveness

- Everyone has sinned and needs God's forgiveness. Romans 3:23: "All have sinned and fall short of the glory of God."
- God's forgiveness is in Jesus only. Ephesians 1:7: "In Him we have redemption through His blood, the forgiveness of our trespasses, according to the riches of His grace."

A Is for Available

- God's forgiveness is available for all. John 3:16: "God loved the world in this way: He gave His One and Only Son, so that everyone who believes in Him will not perish but have eternal life."

- God's forgiveness is available but not automatic. Matthew 7:21: "Not everyone who says to Me, 'Lord, Lord!' will enter the kingdom of heaven."

I Is for Impossible

- According to the Bible, it is impossible to get to heaven on our own. Ephesians 2:8-9: "By grace you are saved through faith, and this is not from yourselves; it is God's gift—not from works, so that no one can boast."

So how can a sinful person have eternal life and enter heaven?

T Is for Turn

- If you were going down the road and someone asked you to turn, what would he or she be asking you to do? Change direction. Turn means repent. Turn away from sin and self. Luke 13:3: "Unless you repent, you will all perish as well!"
- Turn to Jesus alone as your Savior and Lord. John 14:6: "I am the way, the truth, and the life. No one comes to the Father except through Me."
- Here is the greatest news of all. Romans 10:9-10: "If you confess with your mouth, 'Jesus is Lord,' and believe in your heart that God raised Him from the dead, you will be saved. With the heart one believes, resulting in righteousness, and with the mouth one confesses, resulting in salvation."

What happens if a person is willing to repent of his sins and confess Christ?

H Is for Heaven

- Heaven is a place where we will live with God forever. John 14:3: "If I go away and prepare a place for you, I will come back and receive you to Myself, so that where I am you may be also."
- Eternal life begins now with Jesus. John 10:10: "I have come that they may have life and have it in abundance."

H Can Also Stand for How

How can you have God's forgiveness, eternal life, and heaven? By trusting Jesus as your Savior and Lord. You can do this right now by praying and asking Jesus to forgive you of your sins and inviting Jesus into your heart.

Accepting Christ is just the beginning of a wonderful adventure with God! Get to know Him better in a number of ways:

- Follow Christ's example in baptism.
- Join a church where you can worship God and grow in your faith.
- In your church, get involved in Sunday school and Bible study.
- Begin a daily personal worship experience with God, where you study the Bible and pray.[4]

---

[4] www.lifeway.com/Article/Salvation-Through-Christ-A-Matter-of-FAITH

Made in the USA
Middletown, DE
08 July 2018